CYNTHIA ROWLAND

FACIAL MAGIC
The Natural Way to an Ageless Face

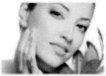
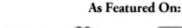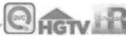
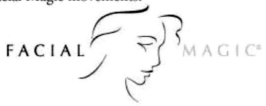

Facial Magic®

Rediscover the Youthful Face You Thought You Had Lost Forever!

Save Your Face with 18 Proven Exercises
to Lift, Tone and Tighten
Sagging Facial Features

Book cover by Lisa Kendrick and interior design by Kali Browne.

Published by:
Rejenuve, Inc.
P.O. Box 549
Newalla, OK 74857
www.cynthiarowland.com

ISBN 978-0-9883742-1-8
Printed in the United States of America

DISCLAIMER
This health information is solely for educational purposes and is not intended to replace your physician nor is it a prescription of medical advice. Application of this information is at the reader s own risk; this information is intended to be discussed with reader s physician to determine the appropriateness and applicability. If you have a pre-existing medical condition or are currently under a physician s care or are taking medication, do not change or discontinue the recommendations of your physician without his/her knowledge. Take this book to the doctor with you.

Table of Contents

Acknowledgements...

So many people have touched my life, believing in my vision to bring this information to all who want to capture the fountain of youth.

Howard Harmon who has provided such incredible support, helping me maintain my vision while working every spare moment to assure that this book was constructed in a timely manner. Thank you for providing me with many wonderful years of friendship and companionship.

Marcia Devon, a wonderful friend and very fine lawyer who keeps my feet on the ground and my head out of the clouds with her sage advice.

Marlene Hartsman, the "sassiest" woman I know who suggested years ago that I write this book and held my hand throughout the summer when I actually wrote it commiserating with me when I could not go to Paris.

Nina Nichols, a long-time friend who always makes me laugh. Her beauty is astounding and her love for life is infectious.

Jackie Silver, my Ageless Sister, BFF and cheerleader. I appreciate you! I adore you!

Steven Tassopoulos, many thanks to you for holding my hand and keeping me sane throughout the years with lots of love and laughter.

Foreword: Testimonial from Marlene Hartsman

Ladies and gentlemen, you have just made one of the most important purchases you will make in your lifetime! I have the pleasure of introducing you to Cynthia Rowland. Cynthia taught me all about Facial Magic in 1994 while we were both doing shows on a home shopping network. I wish you could see the face that I saw – young and gorgeous (I wish I had her nose) with skin that was flawless and radiant. I was with my sister and we both thought Cynthia was in her late 20's or early 30's. As the day unfolded and we all traded stories, Cynthia shared with us the fact that she was almost 47!!! I thought boy, she must have a great plastic surgeon and I wished I was not such a chicken!

Right now I am going to tell you something that will make your day. You are 6 weeks away from seeing miracles! Do not be skeptical. This is going to work for you just like it has for hundreds of thousands of women and men around the world.

All you need is a 9-week commitment (there is that "c" word)-that is all you will need to be a Facial Magic user for the rest of your life!

Let me ask you something simple. When you want to try and get a washboard stomach, you buy an "ab" exerciser. Right? Or if you want to tighten your "tush", do you smear cream all over it, go to bed and wake up the next morning expecting results? Of course not! If there were such a cream, this book would be about that instead! What you and everyone else does is EXERCISE!!! Well, here is the good news. Your face will tighten and the lines and sagging chin will respond to exercise. More good news! The muscles in your face will respond quickly as you perform these very specific, very targeted exercises. Can you stand just one more bit of good news? The exercises are simple. You do not have to put on workout clothes, or even work up a sweat. Facial Magic takes only minutes a day. (I bet you peeked at the "before" and "after " photos before you bought this book – so keep in mind those people got those results in about 15 minutes a day).

Facial Magic is a program that was developed and used in a clinic in Denver about 13 years ago. Women came to this clinic to learn the Facial Magic techniques. They paid $1100.00 each and nobody left disappointed. This program is thorough and unique. It works! Just put in the effort and you will get the results.

No more worrying about birthdays! When you look wonderful it can and will affect all aspects of your life – including your self-confidence and your self-esteem.

In this crazy world where it seems everything is out of control, here is something that you *can* control!

So, I would like to now introduce you to Cynthia Rowland, my friend and my teacher.

Turn the page and let THE MAGIC BEGIN!!!!!!!

MARLENE CORISTINE HARTSMAN
TORONTO, ONT. CANADA

Introduction

Hello, my name is Cynthia Rowland, and I am the creator of Facial Magic, the facial exercise program that has changed hundreds of thousands of faces across the globe.

I learned of this exercise program when my friend Taylor called from Denver to say that she had discovered a small clinic that specialized in **natural facelifts**.

You know how we talk with our girlfriends about the latest and greatest crazes. Whether it's hemlines or lip lines, the newest color trends for a particular season or just how we can improve ourselves, we discuss lots of topics in depth. That's how I learned that my sagging left eyelid would not require surgical intervention.

In one of our many telephone conversations, I was lamenting to Taylor that "practically overnight" my left eyelid had found a new home; it was resting on my eyelash! I hated that look because instantly it made me look tired but most of all, it made me look old.

Spending thousands of dollars in surgery fees did not excite me. Recovery, risk, *surprises,* and pain is not for me; however, my choices to deal with my sagging eyelid were actually very slim. Surgery was the only thing I knew.

But exercise for the face? Would it work for me? Honestly, I had my doubts and I was very skeptical. It was difficult to believe what Taylor was saying.

Taylor convinced me that I should immediately come to Denver. I hoped she was on to something but I had my reservations because it seemed unlikely that if something so wonderful was available, why had I not read about it in the news?

I am glad I flew to Denver to see with my own eyes the results of an exercise program that really, really works. Taylor personally took me to the clinic to meet the staff and I was intrigued from the beginning. People dressed in professional attire passionate about their work, promoting better health with something new: Facial Fitness.

The staff introduced me to women from all walks of life who were willing to show me their before photos. It was evident to me that their faces were indeed different! I could easily see lifting and toning in their faces. I was terribly excited and wanted to learn the exercises myself! Right then!

I stayed in Denver and worked daily at the clinic for over a year to learn how isometric exercise and resistance training can indeed re-shape and contour faces. It was an amazing time for me and I knew that these exercises deserved to be available for everyone, especially because my face began to look younger and younger. And my eyelid? In just weeks, it was much improved and so was my mood!

Did I mention I was forty?

Now, fast-forward ten years: In 1998, the exercise program became available through a worldwide infomercial and the process became the system, **Facial Magic**.

I love sharing the knowledge of keeping your face fit and hope you enjoy this book. The video system provides detailed information and by writing this book, it allows me to enhance the information in a more comprehensive manner.

The Facial Magic regimen is fantastic for restoring muscle tone to your face and neck. You know the look: no matter how much rest you have had, you still "look" tired. Strange things have begun happening to your face. It has begun moving in a Southerly direction and hollows and elevations have begun to develop practically overnight.

You may look into the mirror someday and wonder, "*what happened* to that face I used to know? *How* and when did the drooping and sagging develop and what can I do to stop it?"

It seems to me that the day you discover facial aging is when your "Bad hair days" begin. You have done everything you can do topically, cleansing, moisturizing, exfoliating and yet you see Mother Nature taking her toll – time marching across your face and it is beginning to look old.

Muscles in your face can elongate up to 50% by the time you reach your mid-fifties, so is it any wonder that you wear pools on your jaw line and have droopy upper eyes that make you look tired when you feel so young inside? Your face, the first thing people see, can blatantly shout that you are wearing the ravages of stress, gravity and atrophy. You can cleverly disguise your body with long jackets, black slimming pants, etc, but your face is different. Unfortunately, you cannot mask facial sagging with a new hairdo, makeup or special creams.

Age is not usually bothersome; it is aging that can be almost overwhelming. Is it possible to do something short of surgery to correct those unwanted lines and the underlying problem of muscle atrophy?

FACIAL MAGIC®

You are sophisticated. You know that "miracle creams" can certainly smooth out lines temporarily but there is only one way to non-surgically correct the aging process that results in sagging muscles that create lines and wrinkles, and that is exercise. FACIAL EXERCISE!

Facial Magic is a facial exercise program designed to enhance your appearance and give you great confidence. How you ask? When you take charge of your face, you give yourself the opportunity to restore the toned, lifted look you had when you were younger! When you feel positive about your appearance, I know you will have greater confidence in yourself.

There are added benefits to this program such as better posture and improved skin tone. With Facial Magic you can exercise those hidden muscles and drop years from your face easily, without going to a gym or buying special workout clothing.

I cannot promise that you will look twenty again, however, if you want to drop ten to fifteen years from your face in the next three months and change the shape and contour of your face, you will first need to increase the strength in the muscles underneath the skin. After a few short weeks of exercise, your face will take on a fresh, improved look.

You are never too old or too young to participate in this program. Just as you appreciate the good feelings in your leg and arm muscles when you leg lift, weight train, run or bicycle, the muscles in your face respond the very same way. Your face will feel revitalized and refreshed from the very first day you begin this program!

Facial muscles are much smaller than most muscle groups and experience tells me they rehabilitate easily. Every woman and man that I have personally supervised has received very pleasing results using Facial Magic. Most muscles in the face are attached to skin and this program will teach you how to successfully manipulate these muscles so that you will achieve a more youthful face. Your skin will become vibrant and healthy looking, too.

Since Facial Magic introduces two exercises at a time your muscles strengthen slowly yet deliberately. In a few weeks, you will be working all areas of your face and neck and experiencing a toned, contoured and a lifted appearance.

Resistance training and isometric contractions will produce smoother skin and a healthier glow. This is achieved from increased oxygen and blood supply to the facial area reducing puffiness due to edema (excess water accumulation) as well as hollowness and other symptoms of muscle atrophy.

The Facial Magic program is **natural, safe and easy.** Usually, results are seen immediately! As you perform these exercises, you will see your face change: lines and wrinkles will appear smoother and your eyes will seem more open and you will appear less tired.

When you first begin the program, you will see and feel definite changes in the upper eye and upper cheek areas. The effect is immediate. These changes are temporary and your face will return to its original position, BUT NOT FOR LONG! Regular exercise will result in more permanent changes. Very pleasing results are visible in a few short weeks!

Facial atrophy causes muscles to shift, thus dragging the skin in ways that either reveal your age or exaggerate it. Facial Magic teaches you how to contract your facial muscles through a special anchoring technique. You will learn how to create a contraction by using your fingers to artificially anchor the muscles. This special anchoring is required so that your face responds to the exercises.

Each exercise you learn requires thirty-five seconds. Fifteen to twenty minutes per day is all you need to *complete* all of your exercises. In the beginning two or even four exercises will not consume the allotted time, but gradually, as you memorize each movement, you will discover that the complete basic program can be accomplished in less time than you thought possible.

The old adage, "practice makes perfect" is certainly true of any type of exercise but especially for Facial Magic. The first few times you attempt a new exercise, you may wonder if you are executing it correctly. This book will thoroughly explain each exercise and the exact placement of your hands and fingers. Do you remember learning to drive a car or play tennis or master a golf swing? The actions that seem so automatic now were all somewhat awkward and time consuming at first. Learning the exercises will probably feel the very same way.

Since you look at your face daily, gradual changes may not be apparent to you. That is why I insist that pictures be taken **before** you begin this program. Take three close-up photos, one of each side of your face and a frontal view as well. If you want to print them, there is special area for you to paste your before photos in your workbook. If you want to leave them in your phone until you have reached your fifteenth week of Facial Magic that is okay, too. Just get the photos taken and take them again at the end of every third week: Take "before" pictures on day one of Week One, more at the end of Week Three, new sets at the ends of Week Six, Week Nine, Week Twelve, and the last set at the end of Week Fifteen.

Most users of the video portion of the Facial Magic system have told me in their own words with their accompanying photos, that *they look at least ten years younger* in nine to twelve weeks of performing the Facial Magic exercises! They are thrilled that their faces have become firmer and lifted.

This book will provide you with a very valuable system to take control of your face. Facial Magic will show you how to counteract gravity and sagging, while helping you sculpt your new look.

Your face will feel energized as it benefits from the increased oxygen and blood flow that occurs with the movements. The muscles will respond positively. You will feel refreshed and renewed every day.

Now begin to create a love affair with your face.

Chapter One – From the Inside Out...Affirmations

True beauty begins on the inside; your thoughts, your words and actions portray who you really are.

Affirmations have always been so empowering for me and throughout the years I have repeated many of them over and over again. As you begin the rejuvenation process, you are going to be staring at yourself in the mirror, getting to know your face better and better. The exercises require strict attention and this is the perfect time to begin saying positive things about yourself and your life.

Saying them aloud is a freeing experience. If you have never used affirmations, you will find that verbalizing them gives them great power. As you repeat your affirmations daily, you will discover that they easily come to mind when stressful situations arise or when you feel particularly good, or when you need to lift your spirits.

Each chapter will include affirmations that will help you to become more courageous, stronger and wiser in whatever you set your mind to do. As you continue to repeat the affirmations, they will help you draw on unlimited strength and understanding.

Our minds are connected to our bodies. Our bodies are connected to our minds. Sometimes we say the most negative things to ourselves when we are angry, frustrated or fearful. All these derogatory things that we call ourselves can be stored in a sub-conscience tape that seems to play when we are feeling low. These messages can contribute to low self-esteem and it is my aim to help you move forward with your life so that you are a more positive and upbeat person. Affirmations will help you to be in a place of power.

When you say an affirmation you are stating or asserting positive messages that, even in the face of all contrary evidence, can bring a desire into being. Just wait for the Universe to perform and fulfill.

The use of affirmations sets up change. There is a saying that goes, "Our thinking makes it so." Dwelling on the good will help you to become more loving and when one is loving and kind, everything seems to work better.

Our first affirmation:
Every day, in every way, I am better and better.

Chapter Two – Creating the Look & the Life You Want

There are a number of ways to help you look your best and feel on top of your game. Nutrition, vitamin therapy, sleep, rest, meditation, exercise, water, breathing, walking. You get the idea. All are important aspects to the overall good health and well-being we seek.

Most of the things you ingest show on your face. Too much salt, sugar, or alcohol can produce under eye puffiness and edema in your face.

Did you know that water is designed to flush the system? Drinking more water will promote better health. We will address this in the Water and Oxygen chapter.

For you to have the very best experience with Facial Magic you may have to rethink certain eating patterns and lifestyles. This program of facial health has evolved over many years and a great deal of information has been gathered which is vitally important to your success with Facial Magic.

"Exercise is the Fountain of Youth" says Jackie Silver, founder and creator of Aging Backwards and AgingBackwards.com

There is nothing better than to feel absolutely terrific about yourself. When you feel good, you are radiant, and exude confidence. People are attracted to you simply from the confidence you have in yourself.

Facial Magic will help you become more secure in your appearance. "Bad hair days" will become a thing of the past. As you exercise and gain more and more control, your life can become more enjoyable. Facial Magic will restore a more youthful look that will be observed by all who see you.

It is important to clear your thoughts so that new ideas can spring forth. It is crucial that you set aside time each day for yourself so that you can concentrate on the movements you are performing and just be still. Facial Magic will feel like a pampering session every day. Pampering is something all of us need daily because we typically give so much of ourselves to others that we sometimes forget that we need quiet, personal time, too.

As you develop this love affair that begins with your face, you will experience renewed vitality and enjoy a more youthful appearance. Your life will become more enriched and you will look and feel more alive with each passing day.

"I am happy, I am healthy, I am prosperous!"

Chapter Three – Learning the Basics, our ABC's

To effectively perform this exercise program, there are hints and tips to make your experience easy and enjoyable. Some of these tips are just common sense; others are nuggets that have been passed around the beauty community for a very long time.

Exercising with Facial Magic is your quiet time. It is important that you choose a time of day for performing your exercises when you are relaxed and undisturbed. Your full concentration on each movement will assure that you are performing it correctly and that the maximum benefit is gained each time.

Make certain your face is clean. If you choose to perform your exercises in the morning after your shower or bath, wash your face in the shower and pat it dry. Some of you may need to lightly moisturize your face if you feel that your skin is dry or taut. If you choose to perform the exercises before bedtime, wash your face, hold off using a moisturizer unless your face feels taut and perform the movements required.

Always perform your exercises in front of a mirror. You may sit or stand, whichever is more comfortable for you. Performing each movement in front of a mirror allows you to constantly examine your face to make certain you are not squinting or wrinkling any area while performing the exercise.

All exercises should be performed six (6) consecutive days a week. <u>Exercise once a day.</u> Do not perform the exercises on the seventh day, as this is a day of rest for your face. I usually reserve Sunday as my "rest day".

Each exercise of your program requires four repetitions. The first repetition is held for five (5) seconds, followed with three consecutive repetitions of ten (10) seconds each. Between each repetition, remove your hands from your face and take a deep cleansing breath so that you expand your diaphragm. Exhale through your nose. Do not wait longer than ten to fifteen seconds before resuming the exercise repetition.

It is imperative that you focus on the particular muscle group that is being exercised. Refer often to the facial muscle line drawings along with the musculature diagram that accompanies each exercise. Keep the rest of your body relaxed. Your mind and your muscles need to work together.

Clear your thoughts while exercising and concentrate on each step. You will be delighted by how emotionally relaxed and physically toned you will feel.

Gradually tense the muscles with careful and deliberate movements. The same principles apply to facial exercises as to exercises for other parts of your body. Slow and steady movements firm the face faster than quick, jerky actions.

When performing the exercises that require you to work both sides of your face simultaneously, be certain to apply <u>even</u> pressure to both sides. During the first week or two of the program do not exercise too vigorously. The muscles and skin build slowly. As in other types of exercise, your goal is to build, strengthen and contour.

If some lines and wrinkles seem to be accentuated while you are performing the exercises, you may need to reposition your fingers. Positioning is very important and correct placement of the hands and fingers is imperative to your success. Try not to aggravate existing wrinkles and lines while performing your exercises. If you find that wrinkles are accentuated, begin the movements again and reposition your fingers until you are certain that you are not creating a line or wrinkle in your face.

Always scrutinize the position of your hands and your features in the mirror. Even after you are familiar with every movement, it is important to recheck your hand and face positions from time to time, and to review the exercises in this book.

Do not forget to breathe! Breathe deeply and frequently while performing your exercises. Your muscles need the extra oxygen to revitalize and brighten your face!

Mother Nature works slowly but surely. Experience with clients has helped me to estimate the time needed for your "lift" and other specific results. Learning the initial program in nine weeks requires your dedication. Exercising your face six days a week for fifteen weeks will create a dramatic improvement in skin tone, elasticity, firmness and overall lifting.

Do not rush. Take the time needed to learn each movement correctly. Follow the step-by-step method prescribed for each exercise and **do them in the order they are written**. Make certain you are totally comfortable with each movement before you execute it.

Become aware of your facial posture. Frowning, squinting, pursing your lips, and other contortions of the face will take their toll over the years. If you are game, place a mirror on your desk where you can watch yourself for an entire eight hours. I think you will be surprised by how many times you catch yourself frowning and squinting. There is an easy remedy for frowning: when you feel a frown coming on, gently touch the area between your eyebrows to relax the area.

The same goes for wrinkling your forehead. Just by touching your forehead with your ring finger until the area is relaxed will stop the frowning.

Most vertical frown lines need special attention at night. If you concentrate daily by knitting your brows together, most likely you make the very same motion at night when you are sleeping. To help alleviate the stress on this area at night place a small piece of transparent tape over the area between your eyebrows so that the motion cannot be made. These "concentration" lines are actually a form of frowning. The appearance of these one or two vertical lines can create questions such as "Are you angry?" "Did I say something that upset you?" So, become aware of them NOW! There is a special exercise just for those pesky little lines that will strengthen the area and as you become more aware of the motion that creates them, they will become less apparent. Believe it or not, the tape will not allow you to frown in your sleep!

One Facial Magic user took my suggestion of using the transparent tape on her vertical forehead lines and was very pleasantly surprised by the results. She was so elated that she wrote to say that she now uses transparent tape horizontally on her forehead and around her mouth while she sleeps to keep her face free of contortions.

> *When sleeping and when you are alone, place a one inch piece of "office tape" **vertically** over the 11's in your forehead.*

Chapter Four – Sleep and Your Sleeping Positions

Sufficient sleep is essential for restoration and stress release. So many times, women will complain that they see wrinkles appearing out of nowhere and they are not too happy to see these annoying little lines and creases come to visit.

Recently, a woman friend was complaining that even though she was a faithful Facial Magic user, little lines and creases were showing up every morning. My first thought was that her sleeping position was creating these creases so I asked her to lie on her bed and demonstrate her favorite sleeping posture. Just as I suspected, the position of her face on her pillow was creating lines.

Now ladies, sleep lines are very cute on a three year old but they are not welcomed on our faces!

We spend hours each day sleeping. This is good. Rest relaxes us and allows us to restore ourselves. Getting at least seven hours of sleep per night will not only alleviate stress but will aid in healing. It has been my experience that many of us sleep incorrectly and this can be easily remedied.

Facial Magic strengthens your facial muscles and improves your skin tone.

Elevate your headboard

Take two old phone books, at least one to two inches thick, and place one under each foot of the headboard of your bed. You probably will not notice a difference when you are sleeping but the added elevation will help under eye drainage and help to alleviate under eye puffiness.

Use a Buckwheat Pillow

Perhaps you have heard of the buckwheat pillow. It is a pillow filled with buckwheat hulls that properly aligns your head and neck with your body. This little wonder also helps keep your head cool while you are sleeping and most importantly, it keeps your face from wrinkling! Sleeping on a "bucky" also keeps your head better elevated so that lymph drainage is increased. My friend reported that after a few nights of sleeping on her "bucky", she awoke with no lines on her face or forehead.

Sleeping on a too flat pillow means that fluid and fat can accumulate in your under eye area. Perhaps you have thought that a good night's sleep will make you look more refreshed, yet it hasn't produced the desired results. Most likely, your pillow is the culprit. If your head is not elevated, your under eye area can "bulge", especially if you have eaten overly salty food or enjoyed adult beverages.

If you are unable to find a buckwheat pillow, try sleeping with your pillow tucked behind your ear. This will stop the constant creasing of your face and is especially necessary when sleeping on your side. It is very important for you to position the pillow behind your ear and move it when you turn.

The buckwheat pillow is my personal favorite. Not only is your head cooler at night, the elevation of your head is ideally aligned with your spine and you just cannot create a line or wrinkle on your face when sleeping on this pillow. If you switch to a "bucky," make certain that you lie first on your back with the pillow below your shoulders to align your spine with your head and neck.

Moderate sodium intake

Eye puffiness is usually a result of water retention caused by too much processed salt in the diet and not enough water. Read the labels of everything you ingest and watch for the sodium content. If it is high, eat or drink less of it and see if you experience improvement. If you choose a can of soup and the sodium content is 870 milligrams, put it back. That is high sodium content. Most packaged foods will contain much higher levels of sodium than foods in their natural state.

Sleeping position

Please do not sleep on your stomach – ever! This sleeping position can manifest lower back problems and it will contribute to small vertical lines on either side of your nose. Not pretty!

Sleeping 7-8 hours on your face for years and years will produce many wrinkles on your forehead and creases in your face. Be aware of how you sleep. Take a mirror with you to your bedroom. Lie on your pillow in your favorite sleeping positions. What does your mirror tell you? Can you see where you are creasing your face? Can you reposition yourself to alleviate the creasing motion? When you find that position where wrinkling is not occurring, tell yourself that this is the ideal sleeping position. I believe your subconscious can help you to sleep night after night so that you are not creating wrinkles on your face. Clear your thoughts, say your prayers and slip into dreamland!

I am a positive influence!

Chapter Five – Water & Oxygen

Drinking water is very beneficial to your overall health and it has been known to alleviate a host of ills.

When someone complains about feeling lethargic, of lower back pain or depression, it is an indication that there is probably insufficient water intake on a daily basis.

If your complexion doesn't appear clear, if you suffer from arthritis or neck pain, it would be of benefit to you to increase your water intake. Perhaps you suffer from extensive dry skin. This may be an indication that too little water is in your system. Most women with beautiful skin drink at least sixty-four ounces of water daily. Wrinkles cannot form easily when your body is hydrated from within.

Sodas and teas are not a substitute for water

Maybe you have been dieting and substituting the recommended eight to ten glasses of water per day with non-caloric soft drinks. Your weight loss may be minimal and you are now tempted to stop the eating plan. Just know that soft drinks do not count as water because the brain and body are able to distinguish what you are drinking.

Sodas, coffee, and tea are not part of the food category. Water is the component our bodies need to *flush toxins* from our systems on a continual daily basis.

Water is considered the most essential nutrient for your good health. Without it you are sluggish, depressed and probably not working at your best. Consider a car's engine. Would you run your car without antifreeze? Would you allow the water to drop to a dangerously low level and endanger the motor? The body can go weeks without food but only days without water. So, drink your eight to ten glasses every day.

64 Ounces per day

It is recommended that we consume at least sixty-four ounces of water per day to keep our bodies operating at optimum health. Just drinking sips all day long does not produce the desired flushing effect as does drinking a large, full glass of water at one time. Yes, you are going to make more restroom visits initially but after a while, your body will compensate for the additional fluid and you will find that you are making fewer trips as the days and weeks progress. If you find repeated trips to the restroom during the night a nuisance, stop drinking water at 6:00 p.m. Just make certain that you drink the required amount of water per day so that you are properly hydrated.

Some women complain of constant constipation. If you suffer from constipation, drink more water. Not only does water stimulate your circulation and elimination process, it regulates and controls the natural moisture balance of your skin.

We have many water choices: Bottled water, filtered water, tap water, treated water, flavored water, etc. Filtered water seems to win in the race for purity. Remember, tap water usually has dehydrating chemicals and minerals that are not very healthy when ingested. If you can install a water filtration system on your main drinking water source, you have taken a major step toward better health.

> *Drink more water. Try for 64 ounces each day. Your skin will thank you for the extra hydration.*

Chug to flush

Just how does one begin the process of introducing sixty-four ounces of water when it has not been part of a beauty regime until now? Grab a bottle of water and "chug". Granted, it is not very lady like but you will be amazed how much water you will drink when it is in a bottle. If you are in an office, keep the bottle on your desk. When you make a restroom trip, take your water bottle and refill it from the water cooler. Keep track in your workbook of how many ounces you drink daily and how many trips to the restroom you make. You will notice that in a few days you are drinking the water with fewer visits to the restroom.

Your body will thank you. Your energy level will increase and you will feel healthier because drinking water is a great first step for creating a new you!

Here are some interesting facts regarding water that I think you will enjoy:

1. 75% of Americans are chronically dehydrated.

2. In 37% of Americans, the thirst mechanism is so weak that it is often mistaken for hunger.

3. Even MILD dehydration will slow down one's metabolism as much as 3%.

4. One glass of water will shut down midnight hunger pangs for almost 100% of the dieters studied in a University of Washington study.

5. Lack of water, the #1 trigger of daytime fatigue.

6. Preliminary research indicates that 8-10 glasses of water a day could significantly ease back and joint pain for up to 80% of sufferers.

7. A mere 2% drop in our body's water can trigger fuzzy short-term memory, trouble with basic math, and difficulty focusing on the computer screen or on a printed page.

8. Drinking 5 glasses of water daily decreases the risk of colon cancer by 45%, plus it can slash the risk of breast cancer by 79%, and one is 50% less likely to develop bladder cancer.

Breathing

Increasing your daily intake of water and incorporating better breathing practices will dramatically improve your facial appearance. When you perform the Facial Magic exercises, you will be asked to breathe. The best breaths are "relaxed belly breaths", the breaths that are taken in through the nose to the diaphragm. You will feel the diaphragm and the lower belly expand as you deeply inhale into your lower belly. The breath is then exhaled through your nose. Practice this beneficial exercise until it feels completely natural to you.

The relaxed belly breaths cleanse you, relax you, and relieve stress. I think a cleansing breath after each repetition is needed so that you stay focused on the muscle group being exercised.

As you progress through the exercises, you will want to contract the abdominal muscles as you exhale through your nose. Just tighten the abdominal wall every time you exhale. Soon you will develop an awareness of contracting the abs when you deeply exhale.

According to medical sources there are a multitude of conditions and diseases that relate to incorrect breathing, and optimal breathers rarely get sick.

Remember, breathing in a relaxed yet deep manner can alleviate stress and tension, helping you to stay focused and feel more energetic.

I am renewed with every breath!

Facial Exercise:
The Natural Way to an Ageless Face.

*Try the World's **BEST-SELLING** Facial Exercise Program.*
*Over **1,000,000** Customers.*

We want to send you your **free gloves** right away, so you can promptly begin our program.

After a few weeks of exercise you will be eligible to participate in a **free** online training class!

Contact Karen@cynthiarowland.com and she will **immediately** send your exercise gloves.

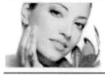

Get the Look of a Facelift Without Surgery!

As Featured On:

    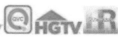

Are You Concerned That Your Face Is *Sagging*?

Even if you are meticulous with your skin care regimen, it's inevitable that your face will start looking tired, and start sagging and becoming elongated as your skin loses its firmness and its youthful contour.

The Facial Magic Exercise regimen requires that exercise gloves be used to execute the Facial Magic movements.

FACIAL 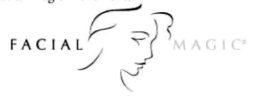 MAGIC®

Other Products Available At:
www.cynthiarowland.com

- **DVD Kits**
- **Free Class**
- **Exercise Gloves**
- **Skin Care Products**
- **Luscious Lips™ Lip Pump**
- **Free Gloves (send e-mail)**

You must register in order to participate.

Don't forget to take beginning photos!

Chapter Six – Diet and Nutrition

Your eating plan

Good nutrition begins with a good eating plan. Raw fruits and raw vegetables contain those all important anti-aging agents that help retard free radicals, the nasty little "PacMen" that wreak havoc on our cells. Medical research has determined that vitamin rich foods may allow you to grow older without growing ill.

More and more we hear about the dangers of excessive sugar and GMO's in our diet. Sugar, white carbohydrates and starches are also smidgens that show on our faces as unwanted fat accumulates. After a while, the effects of fat begin to show in all parts of our bodies. We are at risk of heart disease and a host of other illnesses. Our faces are just like the rest of our bodies. They show weight gain and the effects of junk food. What we eat can sometimes reveal or accentuate our age!

Whatever your weight, height, or body structure, Facial Magic will work for you. After all, you are dealing primarily with muscle and tissue and you will see changes even if you are over your ideal weight by 50 pounds or more.

Body weight

I will let you in on a secret: Most women automatically lose weight when they practice Facial Magic! Something happens when you look at yourself in your mirror everyday. A connection to self develops. You begin to create a love affair and that feeling of love begins to permeate other facets of your life, including how you feel about yourself. As you begin to see overwhelming results with Facial Magic, the good feelings take hold as you take control of the areas in your life that may have been troubling you.

There is a certain confidence that develops when you begin to allow change in your life. When you see your face becoming less lined and stressed, more vibrant and alive, you take those good feelings and apply them to other areas you want to improve.

When you spend time with the before and after photos in this book, you will see women of all ages and shapes who have rehabilitated their faces with this program. Some have lost weight; some have not. But overall, they are more confident in their appearance because they look and feel more comfortable with themselves.

Yes, most of them have adopted a healthier lifestyle and care more about the types of food they use for fuel and for comfort. They have learned that eating raw vegetables and fruits provide them greater vitamin therapy. They have chosen a better lifestyle and they feel more balanced. They learn to eat for health.

Fight free radicals

Some foods that I personally recommend to boost nutrition, increase energy levels and naturally contain anti-aging properties are those full of Vitamin C, A or Beta Carotene and Vitamin E. These foods fight free radical damage. Free radicals roam around in our bodies. They cause severe damage to cell structure that can eventually result in disease.

Foods that naturally contain beta-carotene are dark yellow and vibrant green. They include fruits and vegetables such as apricots, kiwi, mango, papaya, broccoli, cantaloupe, carrots, pumpkin, spinach, squash and sweet potatoes.

Colorful, organic vegetables and fruit – red, yellow, orange and green nourish your body. Eat them raw for healthier looking skin.

Those that naturally contain Vitamin C are asparagus, cauliflower, cabbage, grapefruit, tomatoes, green peppers, red peppers, lemons, potatoes, oranges, parsley and spinach.

Whole grains, vegetable oils, dried beans, peas, and nuts contain Vitamin E.

I encourage you to stop worrying about your weight. Imagine yourself slim and do what slim people do – eat right, eat less and move! During a hypnotherapy session with my girlfriend, Lori, I was given a mantra for keeping in good shape: "I am slim, slim, slim." Repeat it often every day!

There are foods that act as immunity boosters and are important to keep on hand and consume. One is yogurt. Studies have proven that eating six ounces of yogurt per day for at least four months can prevent colds and reduce the symptoms of hay fever.

Another food is garlic. Yes, we have heard how heart healthy individuals proclaim the effects of garlic, but did you know it could also fend off an attack of foreign invaders in your body? Yes! Garlic increases the potency of T-Lymphocytes and macrophages (white blood cells) that protect your immune system.

And don't forget your zinc! This nutrient revitalizes aging immune systems and can speed up the healing of wounds.

I enjoy foods that nourish my body.

Chapter Seven – Exercise and Vitamins

What is it about the idea of exercise that makes it one of the hardest things to commit to for any length of time?

At some time or another, most of us have gotten gung-ho with good intentions and then our schedules create impossible road blocks, providing convenient excuses to stop the exercise regimen.

Move for life

Exercise keeps you alive. Moving is vital to keep you in optimum health. Whether you walk, bicycle, jog, skate, perform martial arts, work out in the gym, or work out at home, all of these activities reward you with better health.

Disease ("dis-ease") is a condition of the body that impairs normal functioning. Disease is a result of lack: lack of exercise, lack of emotional support, lack of water, lack of nutrition…you get the idea. When you make the decision to begin an exercise program, you give yourself a better life. You do not have to wait for months or years to realize the benefits of exercise because it is almost instantaneous.

Lack of physical exercise can result in a host of illnesses that could have possibly been avoided. The benefits of exercise are well documented; just surf the internet and you will see thousands of articles that proclaim exercise is the best way to alleviate heart disease, high blood pressure, back aches and pains, obesity or osteoporosis.

Exercise will increase your endurance and strength. Endurance training, whether it is riding your bicycle, walking or dancing will help build muscle strength that has been lost to disuse. Just as you can see sagging facial muscles, the rest of your body can suffer the very same atrophy. I have seen my thighs jiggle, my bottom begin to slide down my legs and my underarms wave in the breeze, all from a lack of body conditioning and tone.

As you exercise, you are increasing your stamina, your strength, your balance and your bone density.

Getting started

If you are not currently exercising and you are ready to start a new regime, consider walking. Walk around your house, walk down the block, and just begin to move. It is suggested that to begin a 30-minute walking campaign, you only need to walk fifteen minutes away from the house, turn around, and walk home. It is so simple!

With Facial Magic you are taking control of your face and now you can create a better looking, better feeling body. Your legs, your arms, your heart will love the great feelings that are produced and you will feel more alive, centered, and in charge of your health. With regular exercise, like walking or bicycling thirty minutes a day, three times a week, your body will begin to make subtle changes by the third day of exercise. Whether you choose to have fifteen minutes of exercise twice a day, or to complete your outing in thirty minutes, the benefits of feeling better, enjoying life and having more confidence are huge payoffs!

If you have frequent headaches, try walking more and practice your deep breathing techniques. If you feel lethargic, try walking for ten minutes. Your head will clear and you will feel energized.

Facial Magic is safe and easy to learn. Each exercise requires 35 seconds. You will look better and better each day.

Floor exercises

I love "floor exercises" and yoga. I love being on the floor so that I can stretch and perform movements that I learned years ago. The exercises are quick, only twenty minutes a day and they do not produce sore muscles. For years I did not perform any floor exercises, instead, I elected to bicycle, power walk, and weight train. There were also long periods of time when I only walked four blocks to the post office and back to the office.

I discovered that I was walking with shorter steps and I did not feel graceful. My carriage did not seem youthful. I knew I had to be more active. I now perform floor exercises at least three times a week for fifteen to twenty minutes each time. In six weeks, I noticed a steady improvement in my legs and arms. Sit-ups, leg lifts, crunches, stretches, push-ups, give me power and strength. These repetitive movements build stamina and muscle mass. I usually exercise in front of the television set watching a favorite program.

Regular exercise has proven to alleviate a host of ills. You will ward off disease and disability with your new regime and you will look marvelous!

Jack LaLanne method

Jack LaLanne successfully offered stay-at-home moms an opportunity to get in shape using chairs and ottomans as their "equipment". You can do the same. Using the back of a chair, you can do leg extension exercises and calf exercises that will help increase circulation. You can also sit on the chair and work your abs. To tone and condition your arms, you may use an unopened can of peas or green beans as a substitute for a barbell. Turn on the music and dance your way around the kitchen as you prepare dinner, incorporate some yoga moves into your laundry routine. Use your imagination to implement a fitness program right in your own home.

Exercise is really just movement which comes in many forms: walking, yoga, Pilates, dancing, skiing, jogging, bicycling, working out at the gym or at home, any of these activities will reward you with better health benefits. You are increasing your stamina, your strength, your balance and your bone density, all needed in order to age gracefully.

Get a buddy

Build in a social aspect, a walking buddy or swim pal. According to a study done by Michigan State University's, Department of Kinesiology, exercising with a partner can boost your enthusiasm to enjoy and look forward to your workout.

If you have health concerns please check with your doctor before beginning any exercise program, then if you are ready to improve "your everything", get out there and move.

"I honor my body with exercise!"

Chapter Eight – Nutritional Supplements Can Promote Better Health

Vitamin therapy has been big news in recent years. Millions and millions of dollars have been designated for research into the industry of helping people live a better life using vitamin supplements.

In 1968, I began working with the President's First Lady's Health Spa organization that was later headed by Jack LaLanne. In the four years that I worked as a fitness trainer, then manager of these spas, I learned a great deal about supplements to aid in increased energy, anti-aging and protection from disease.

I personally watched Mr. LaLanne gulp down 100+ vitamins at a time! What an eye-opener! This unbelievably fit man was way ahead of his time and he is remembered by everyone for his lifelong commitment to health via exercise and supplements. He believed that an ounce of prevention is worth a pound of cure and so do I.

Many people over the years have asked me about the supplements I take. I am not a physician so please understand that I am speaking from my own personal experience with this vitamin regime that was adopted over thirty years ago. I only ask that you please check with your physician if you have health concerns before running to your nearest vitamin store to buy these preparations.

The majority of my vitamins are taken an hour or so before bedtime. This is an ideal time to take them because by 9:00 p.m., I have mostly digested food in my stomach and I believe this is beneficial to the absorption of the vitamins. Remember, I said the majority. When I prepare my morning power shake at 9:00 – 10:00 a.m. daily, I add ¼ teaspoon Vitamin C crystals so that the absorption rate is accelerated because my stomach is empty. I take no other vitamins in the daytime, just that one small serving of Vitamin C crystals.

Vitamin therapy has been a daily regimen of mine for many years and I continue to enjoy terrific health. In the last five years, I have added Grape Seed Extract and Pycnogenol (50 times more effective as an antioxidant than Vitamin E and 20 times more effective than Vitamin C) to my nightly routine along with Ginkgo Biloba and a super antioxidant mineral formula. Typically, I take the following supplements on a nightly basis:

Supplement	Daily Quantity	Benefit
Grape Seed Extract	150 mg	Improve circulation, antioxidant power
Pycnogenol	recommended	Inflammation fighter, antioxidant power
Alpha Lipoic Acid	200 mg	Increases glutathione, brain function, energy
Astaxanthin	2 gel caps daily	Skin, eye sight, brain function
Pro-biotic - Culturelle	One daily	Fights disease, helps digestion, inhibits bacteria
Gingko Biloba	40 mg	Improve cognitive performance
Vitamin C	3,000 ius daily	Collagen production, prevents cancer
Vitamin E	800 ius daily	Improves skin and hair, anti-aging
Blue/Green Algae (Spirulina)	recommended	Protects from cancer, encourages fat loss
Selenium	200 mcg	Improves immune system
Super Antioxidant Minerals	recommended	Fights free radicals. Reduces inflammation. Enhances skin beauty.
Vitamin D	recommended	Boosts immune system.
B-1	recommended	Supports heart, brain, lungs and kidneys.
Co Enzyme Q-10	200 mg	Supports heart and cell health

I cannot imagine my life without vitamin supplements. I believe they are very important as they can protect us from the environmental damage we experience on a daily basis. I believe that taking supplements daily will help prevent many illnesses.

"Each day I honor my body with good nutrition."

Chapter Nine – Skin Care You Can Count On

There are steps you can take to ensure more beautiful skin. As the Facial Magic exercise system works beneath the skin, it is up to you to enhance your appearance with skin care products that make a difference and application techniques to improve your regimen.

Yes, techniques. Most women and men want to avoid aging, sagging skin and this chapter is dedicated to teaching you how to carefully care for your face. I have seen women scrub their faces like they are scrubbing their kitchen floors. I have even seen models demonstrating products on TV abuse their face with skin stretching techniques. No More! This chapter will help you to understand the importance of gentle actions when caring for your skin. Remember, the goal is to create a love affair with your face.

We have covered water, diet, exercise, vitamins and many other topics in preparation for learning the Facial Magic movements. Now it is time to learn the "straight skinny" on skin care.

Wash your face nightly then use serums, eye cream, treatment and lastly a rich moisturizer

Beware "Natural" skin care

Skin care and color cosmetics are the mainstay of grooming and beauty for women from every culture on the planet. As we have become more sophisticated and educated, we are pretty particular about the types of products we use on ourselves. We've learned that the designation of "natural" doesn't always mean safe (poison ivy is "natural") and cosmetic companies may capitalize on the buzz words du jour like "organic", "green"," botanical", "toxin free", "clean" and probably a few other terms that might actually confuse us.

Today's savvy consumers expect/desire instant gratification from their skin care and beauty products. They also demand long-term results. We like immediate results, but instant gratification means we must wait at least 45 days so that skin turnover will reveal the new skin we crave.

Hazardous chemicals

We rely on the Food and Drug Administration (FDA) to guide our decision making regarding the ingredients in our favorite color cosmetics, hair and skin care products. However, the FDA does not require companies to submit products for review before they market them to us. But consumers are using their voices, and dollars, to say no to harmful ingredients like parabens, mineral oil, glycols, PEGS, hydroquinone, talc, petroleum, synthetic ingredients, carcinogens and phthalates. Some of the up-market companies that manufacture and design cosmetics and toiletries are starting to phase out these types of harmful ingredients, and market the news to consumers to enhance the value of their brand. Until 2013, even Johnson & Johnson Baby Shampoo contained a preservative that released formaldehyde. Why was there a carcinogen in a baby shampoo?

Expensive, dermatologist-recommended and tested or designer cosmeceuticals do not mean toxin or irritation free. Hazardous chemicals are everywhere; some baby shampoos have sulfates which can damage eye tissue, create premature baldness and even cause cataracts. Even toothpaste has harmful ingredients that are not recommended for young ones under the age of six. If you check the toothpaste label, you will read that only a pea-sized amount is suggested for a child. Putting toxic chemicals such as dyes, sugar, fluoride, sodium lauryl sulfate and triclosan in your mouth introduces these substances into your gums and into your blood stream.

When you apply products with toxins topically on your skin – sunscreen comes to mind – these chemicals can penetrate the largest organ of our body – our skin – and head right into our blood stream. Not only that, but many products that are chemically laden promote damage to the very skin we are treating. According to a 2006 study from the University of California, Riverside, certain sunscreen ingredients may cause more free radicals to form than no sunscreen at all.
Not everything is harmful. There are safe products out there. Use your computer or visit a reputable vitamin store to search for the safest, most reliable products for you and your family. Read labels and check your shampoo, toothpaste, lipstick, foundation, mascara, lip & brow lines and skin care product ingredients and educate yourself on the chemicals to avoid.

In a world where we're often judged by how we look, our skin can reveal a lot about us. Smooth, hydrated, glowing skin is a sign of good health. Dry, dull skin makes us look older.

FACIAL MAGIC®

The skin you're in

Most of us take our skin, a most amazing organ, for granted. This remarkable outer covering has many functions that we rarely consider. Our skin holds our muscles, bones and ligaments together, and eliminates toxins through our perspiration, and is a barrier, protecting us from the outside world. Our skin acts as a defense, can alert the body to danger as in OUCH! and can heal itself when traumatized.

The largest organ in your body is your skin, and we need to nourish it by way of exfoliating, cleansing, nourishing and protecting.

Taking you back to your grade school health classes, we learned that our skin is comprised of the epidermis, the outer layer that we see and touch, the dermis, the middle layer where collagen, elastin, blood, hair and sweat glands are and the subcutaneous – the lower level where we find fat and our collagen. The layers of skin are made up of water, lipids, minerals and protein, and all that is packed into a layer 0.5mm thick on your eyelids to 4mm thick on the palms of your hands.

What happens to skin as we age? Well, the skin on our body along with the skin on our face can begin to droop and sag certainly after the age of 40. Collagen production begins to wane, our muscles soften and shrink from disuse and we begin to resemble our elders as we fight our battle with Mother Nature.

Keeping your body at an ideal weight, taking your anti-aging vitamins, drinking plenty of water while enjoying a rich array of colorful veggies every day, will keep your skin taut and healthy looking.

Sun

The sun usually begins damaging our skin at an early age. Even though we love how a tan enhances our appearance, from this day forward it must come from a bottle. Wearing an SPF 15-45 sunscreen will help protect your skin. Even more protection is possible when you include wearing a hat and sunglasses **year round** with your sunscreen. Wearing your sunscreen/sun block year round is recommended because damaging rays not only come from the sun, damaging rays radiate from overhead lighting in the workplace. So, it is imperative that you apply sunscreen to your face, neck, and the back of your neck, chest, and the areas on your arms and legs that are exposed to UV light.

Wrinkling, pigmentation changes, interesting bumps that appear from nowhere and most skin growths are due to sun exposure. We do not like these little surprises when we see them developing on our faces or other parts of our bodies. Most of the changes that we see on our skin, especially those pesky little lines, are not usually the result of aging, but sun damage.

I recently listened to a news story dealing with the use of sunscreen, and I learned that if you continually use sunscreen every day, not only will you likely stop further damage, but you may also lessen the current damage over time. That gives hope to all of us who have sun-damaged skin, so adopt the sunscreen regime now!

My dermatologist and aesthetician friends agree that there are four components that contribute to skin aging: **Sunlight, Gravity, Muscle Movements and Sleeping Positions.**

Sunlight - The biggest culprit is sunlight because it usually creates a very cruel pattern of wrinkles. Sunscreen will dramatically help protect your skin and you are going to win the battle against gravity, muscle movements and sleeping patterns with Facial Magic.

Gravity – An unseen force that pulls towards the earth. In other words, when you look in the mirror and you see telltale signs that your face is elongating, that is the force of gravity. The fold developing near your nose running toward the mouth? Gravity. Your eye makeup is "off" – gravity. You see a slight thickening under your chin – gravity. In fact, most facial muscles will elongate about ½ inch by the age of 55 due to gravity and inactivity of the muscles. We see the effects of gaining ½ inch in our waist, tummy, thighs and hips; our faces show that ½ inch gain as aging.

Muscle Movements – You may be experiencing challenges that affect what I call your facial posture. Do you have frown lines between your eyebrows? Have you noticed that you are smiling less? Surprising as it may seem, a frown requires the use of more muscles than a smile. It only takes 18 muscles to smile and 34 to frown.

Sleeping Positions - When you sleep with your face buried into a pillow, you create wrinkles. Stomach sleepers can expect to see a vertical line develop next to the nose. The forehead may develop diagonal lines near the temples and vertical lines near the ears. Stomach sleepers usually complain of back challenges.

Cleanse, Moisturize, Exfoliate, Protect

These are the components to healthier looking and acting skin. You need synergistic skin care products that are formulated to work together for your skin's maximum benefit.

There have been many breakthroughs in the past few years in the area of skin care. We see Alpha Hydroxy preparations in many strengths; Beta Hydroxy in foams, gel and lotions, Retinoid products, Peptides, Stem Cell and Vitamin C products. There are wrinkle eradicators that are plant based; there are Vitamin E products. The list goes on and on and this list changes all the time. They all have positive effects and can erase years from your face, but how do you choose which will work best for you?

Be consistent with skin care

The advice of dermatologists and aestheticians is to choose one line of products and stay with that line for at least six months so that you have the opportunity to *see results*. If you constantly switch cleansers, occasionally use Vitamin C, use a Retinoid for only a month, you are going to be disappointed because the effects may not be what you expected. In some cases you may have even experienced skin irritations when you were mixing different products. I know I have.

Your skin is endowed by nature with all it requires for optimum health. Age, environmental factors, dietary deficiencies and poor health, all contribute to deplete your skin of natural, vitally important elements.

> *Rubbing your eyes, propping your face or neck in your hands or even stroking or playing with a double chin can adversely affect your skin.*

The Facial Magic Skin Care products, based on peptide technology, are cruelty free products that work to promote a more flawless complexion and they are designed to clean, exfoliate, moisturize and nourish your skin on a daily basis.

While your skin is naturally resilient, the areas of your face and neck demand more attention because they are exposed to the sun, wind, smog, smoke and other pollutants. This over-exposure can cause your face to look dry, wrinkled, or chapped.

Facial Magic provides sensible skin care. It promises to treat your face and complexion with care and reduce fine lines and wrinkles while preventing other signs of pre-mature aging. Remember, everything to which you pay special attention always improves. I cannot think of anything more special than our faces. That is why I will help you with the application of all the products so that your skin will benefit. There is nothing more frustrating than not knowing when to use each product. Should you apply gels first, creams last?

Remember, no one has perfect skin. Mostly everyone I know, including models, actresses and myself have some type of skin challenge. The flawless complexions you see in magazines are the result of airbrushing, not perfect skin.

As we age, our skin becomes dryer and thinner because new cell growth is slower and oil gland function diminishes, resulting in dryness and skin sensitivity. You may feel that you have lost that youthful glow. You will be happy to know that our products address mature skin; skin that is thirsty and crying to be replenished with moisture.

The name of the game is enhancement. In this chapter, you will learn how to exfoliate, cleanse, and pamper your face in the most beneficial ways.

Specific Skin Challenges

Many women have asked me about specific problems relating to their skin and I want to take the opportunity to discuss some of those questions.

Adult Acne and Stress

One perplexing problem we women have to deal with is adult acne. What causes this and how do we correct it?

Those pesky pimples can pop up at the most inconvenient times - right? They can appear just as you are ready to interview for that all important job, and then you know for certain that you are having a "Bad hair day." Perhaps your son or daughter's wedding day is approaching and the stress level is soaring or maybe the reunion is fast approaching and you are still dieting. Whatever!

Your face is always changing in response to what occurs around you, and stress affects the facial skin and the eye area. You may be experiencing challenges that affect your facial posture, i.e., you may discover frown lines between your eyebrows, and you may notice that you are smiling less. (Surprisingly as it may seem, a frown requires the use of more muscles than a smile. It only takes eighteen muscles to smile and thirty-four to frown.) You may find your face changing before your eyes.

FACIAL MAGIC®

You are in for such a satisfying experience when the Facial Magic exercises and the skin care work for you. Many women have expressed how the stress in their faces lifts away and their skin appears clearer and more vibrant when they use my program.

Pimples can show up long after your teenage years. Adult acne, which is more prevalent in women than in men, primarily pops up on chins, jaw lines and necks. Adult acne has the same cause as teenage acne: pores clogged by cells that slough off from the oil ducts in the skin. If the plug comes to the surface at a pore's opening, the result is a blackhead. If it does not manifest as a blackhead, bacteria becomes trapped behind the plug where it feeds on the backed up oil, causing painful inflammation and giant eruptions.

Some of you may notice that acne seems to be concentrated on your chin and along the jaw line. If that is so, please consider how you use your telephone. If you are on the phone a lot and press the handset close to your face, you may be irritating your skin and causing the outbreak. Try swabbing the receiver with alcohol every morning and learn to hold the receiver away from your face rather than resting it between your chin and shoulder. There are some pretty terrific headset phones available that can set your hands free and allow the facial area that has been irritated to heal. Using a headset phone will also relieve neck and shoulder stress. I highly recommend them.

No matter your skin type, keep your hands away from your face! Be aware of your facial posture and wash your face before bedtime.

Rosacea

Sometimes in mature skin, a condition called acne rosacea appears affecting the nose, cheeks, and forehead. The inflammation comes and goes. Often, pimples develop in these areas that become oily and red. After time broken blood vessels can appear and, in extreme cases, the nose can become extremely red and enlarged. There are a host of reasons for rosacea. Please check with your physician if you believe you may have this condition. The National Rosacea Society has a website worth reading, you may access them at: http://www.rosacea.org.

Dry Skin

When your face is overly dry, you may feel a tight, pulling sensation, especially after cleansing and prominent wrinkles or lines may appear on the surface of your skin. Lowering the water temperature in your shower or bath and when you wash your face will lessen the tautness you now experience. More than a lukewarm temperature is taxing to your skin. Cleansing your face with a clean cloth and a ph-balanced cleanser will enhance your skin almost immediately. Try drinking more water and moisturize your face well before retiring.

Unfortunately, dry skin becomes more pronounced as you age. Photo aging (excessive exposure to the sun) can speed up natural changes you see in your face when the cell turnover begins to slow. Results of photo aging can be seen in skin that is losing its resilience earlier than you would like, and the surface texture begins to feel leathery while crisscrossed lines appear on your chin and around your mouth.

Dry skin is known clinically as "Essential Fatty Acid Deficiency." The climate in which you live may also be a contributing factor to your skin's condition because autumn and winter bring dry heat into your home.

Dry skin can show up as red, itchy, flaky skin on your legs, arms, hands and even your face. The best advice is: turn down the heat in your showers and in your home, moisturize your face and body well, use ph balanced cleansers, drink more water and use your sunscreen every day.

Oily Skin

Oily skin usually results in enlarged pores, especially around the nose, and a shiny complexion shortly after cleansing. Skin blemishes may appear on the face and across the shoulders and you may perspire freely. To help alleviate this condition, frequent washing of your face is advised using a ph-balanced facial cleanser. The action of natural ingredients in the cleanser can prevent the production of excessive oil and help maintain clear skin.

The Facial Magic exercise program will assist in eliminating that greasy feeling by increasing oxygenated blood to the tissues. Also, drinking water promotes the body's ability to balance excessive oily skin. So get that water bottle out and drink up!

Let me assure you that properly caring for your face is easy and it doesn't take much time when you know what products work for you. Many women have asked about my daily regimen: When do you do your exercises? What foundation do you use? Do you use your own products? What do you do to keep your face in great shape?

FACIAL MAGIC®

Cynthia's Daytime Regimen for the Face

     1. Facial Magic detergent free Cleanser

     2. Facial Magic facial exercise

     3. Exfoliation using Facial Magic Daily Lift Alpha Hydroxy Gel Mask

     4. Vitamin C Serum

     5. Facial Magic Firm and Repair Peptide Serum

     6. Facial Magic Eye Treatment

     7. Facial Magic Daytime Skin Nutrition

     8. Sunscreen SPF 30

     9. Foundation and makeup

1. Cleansing the Face

Use a Cleansing Gel that is a gentle, detergent free cleanser with foaming lipoproteins that purifies the skin as it deep cleans and retains the natural moisture balance. A good cleanser prepares the skin to receive maximum benefits from the other treatments.

Your face needs to be cleansed twice daily: once in the morning to remove nighttime preparations (this is easily done in the shower) and again before bedtime to remove makeup that was applied during the day.

The benefits of a clean face are many; the goal is to keep bacteria levels that naturally occur to a minimum.

Pull your hair back with a band so that your entire face is exposed.

Pour a pea-sized amount of the cleanser into the palm of your hand and then use the fingertips to apply the gel to your face, neck and upper chest area. Remember; gently apply the product with your fingertips. Let the gel sit on your face, neck and chest for one full minute so that the makeup, dirt, and grime accumulated during the day are dissolved and released.

Now, wet a clean washcloth with lukewarm water and gently remove the gel starting with the chest area first. Rinse and wring the washcloth and begin removing the cleansing gel with soft, upward strokes. Rinse and wring the washcloth with clean lukewarm water before moving to the neck area. **Remember, it is essential to always use a clean washcloth every time you cleanse to ensure that bacteria are not transferred to your skin. Use one washcloth at night and a different one in the morning.**

The skin on your neck is similar to your under eye area and must be handled gently. Use upward and outward strokes with your clean washcloth to remove the residue of the cleanser.

Rinse your washcloth thoroughly.

Next, remove the gel from your face, beginning near your mouth and moving your washcloth out to the hairline. This is an upward and outward movement. Cleanse both sides of your face before moving to your forehead. Rinse your washcloth frequently so that you are removing the gel with clean water.

After the gel has been removed, rinse your face again by splashing lukewarm water on your face, neck and chest area. No scrubbing or rubbing allowed!

Pat the cleansed areas with a clean towel. It is not necessary to completely dry your face, as the moisturizers will help lock in moisture that is already present.

2. Perform the Facial Magic Exercises

3. Apply the Facial Magic Daily Lift Exfoliant (This is a completely unique skin care product that revolutionizes mask treatments)

Create a love affair with your face using Facial Magic to lift, tone and tighten your facial features.

Facial Magic Daily Lift is a purified gel mask containing a proprietary natural complex Alpha Hydroxy Acid with a natural protease extract. Protease is a naturally occurring enzyme, which will help prevent your face from experiencing skin irritation. Our formula has a special dual action: Daily Lift gently removes environmentally damaged skin cells and rejuvenates the skin by producing a smooth and tightened surface. It is designed for use every day, two weeks at a time with a two-week rest period. I recommend that when you begin using this product, you only leave it on five minutes and then after a week of use, leave it on for ten minutes before removing.

This gentle preparation is recommended for the face, neck and chest area and can even be used under the eyes to remove environmentally damaged skin. By using Daily Lift, your skin will be prepared to receive maximum benefits from your moisturizers and the other treatments. Old cells, when allowed to stay on the skin, block the effectiveness of other preparations. Your foundation will glide on effortlessly and your pores will appear more tightened after using Daily Lift. This product is available at www.cynthiarowland.com.

FACIAL MAGIC®

To begin, cleanse your face, pat semi-dry with a clean towel and then gently apply a thin layer of the gel over your face, neck and chest area using light stokes. No pulling or tugging of your skin is allowed. Make certain you do not allow the gel to come in contact with your eyes although you may use this product under your eye area. Allow the gel to stay on for five to ten minutes.

Using a clean, lukewarm, wet washcloth, remove the gel just as you do the cleanser. Beginning with the chest area, remove in soft upward strokes. Rinse the washcloth thoroughly before moving to the neck area.

Remove the Daily Lift from your neck area with soft, gentle, upward and outward movements. Rinse the washcloth and go over the area to make certain that any residue is removed.

Using upward and outward motions, remove the gel from your face moving from your mouth to your hairline area. Rinse the washcloth frequently to ensure complete removal of the gel. Be gentle with your face when removing this product. Run your hands over your skin when you have removed the Daily Lift from your face, neck and chest one last time to make certain that all traces are removed.

4. Applying the Vitamin C Serum

Use a high quality Vitamin C Serum. Vitamin C Serum plumps the skin to reduce the appearance of fine lines and wrinkles as it lightens skin tone and age spots. Vitamin C Serum stimulates skin cell regeneration and the production of collagen, elastin and other important components of the "intercellular matrix" (the layers of your skin).

Pump a few drops onto your fingertips and dot your face, neck and chest area with the Serum. Using gentle, soft, circular strokes, massage the Serum into the skin. As you apply the Serum to your face, massage in an upward, circular motion away from your mouth. After you have massaged the Serum into the skin, wait a few minutes before applying any other preparation so that the penetration is complete. Do not forget to apply the Vitamin C Serum under and around your eyes and onto the back of your hands.

5. Applying the Facial Magic Firm & Repair Peptide Serum

Peptides are the ultimate in better skin care. Peptides are akin to building blocks for the skin and I believe they are important for hydrated, radiant skin, especially facial skin. Peptides help replace lost collagen and by using this remarkable product, the peptides stimulate the synthesis of collagen by more than 300%. In other words, peptides trick the body into producing more collagen.

Pump a few drops onto your fingertips and massage into your skin in upward, circular strokes away from your mouth. Make certain you cover your forehead, neck and face thoroughly and allow your skin to "rest" for at least a minute for maximum absorption before applying the next preparation.

6. Applying the Facial Magic Eye Treatment

You will want to use an eye treatment that offers properties to nourish and condition your under eye tissue. A superior cream transports high performance regenerating ingredients to the area around the eye to reduce the appearance of fine lines and wrinkles. Your eye treatment needs to improve hydration with a cumulative effect, the longer you use it, the better the results.

Your under eye area is prone to extreme dryness due to the body's inability to naturally moisturize this region. This arid condition equates to a dull, lifeless, nutrient starved look.

The best eye treatments offer light diffusing properties that allow immediate results to be seen in your entire eye region. You will notice a smoothing, soothing effect as puffiness and dryness are erased.

Dark circles usually make us appear tired. Those raccoon discolorations can be lightened with continual use of a quality Eye Treatment. Again, increase your water consumption to flush out toxins and impurities in your body.

I recommend application of your Eye Treatment twice daily; once in the morning and again before bedtime. If your eye region is over-exposed to the elements, i.e., sun, wind, harsh light, smog, etc., at any time during the day, by all means, re-apply your Eye Treatment to keep your very delicate eye area moist.

To correctly apply your Eye Treatment, use your ring finger. Why the ring finger? This finger has the least amount of strength and provides the lightest touch. It is the most suitable to use in this delicate region.

Face your mirror. Place the Eye Treatment on each ring finger. Gently "pat" the treatment all around your upper and lower eyes. Then place your fingertips under your inner eyebrows and continue outwards until a full circle has been completed around your upper and lower eye region. Again, slowly begin to move your fingertips outward, then toward the inner corner of the under eye area in a circular motion. Gently perform this "exercise" about 100 times around each eye.

Before you begin, make sure your entire under eye area is sufficiently moisturized. This "exercise" will stimulate the blood flow around your eyes.

7. Applying the Moisturizers

Our Facial Magic Daytime Skin Nutrition ™ (Day Cream) and our Overnight Sensation ™ (Night Cream) are "wrinkle defense" products consisting of deeply penetrating formulas that help reduce the appearance of lines and wrinkles on contact. They are designed to hold the moisture balance of the skin during the day under makeup and at night while you sleep. They act as deep tissue regenerators by retarding the damage caused by free radicals.

The Day Cream and Night Cream contain powerful peptides and anti-oxidants. Red Marine Algae and Biopeptide CL provide skin with the nutrition it needs to fight free radical damage, regenerate anti-oxidants and eliminate damaged collagen to ensure that your skin receives nutrients and protection throughout the day and night.

Protection? Yes, premature aging results from free radicals, toxic substances that are created during a cell's metabolism - its natural life span. Many more free radicals are produced when the body experiences the stresses of everyday life.

Look radiant and de-stressed in just weeks using our facial exercises that will help you look better than you have in years.

Be certain to use the moisturizers daily.

Moisturizers are applied after all of your other skin care treatments. Remember, the facial skin is not required to be dry for the application of the moisturizers, in fact, a slight dampness is recommended. The Eye Treatment is applied before the moisturizers using the method we previously discussed.

Rule of thumb: be sure to cover every area of your face, neck and chest with the moisturizing creams so that your skin is well hydrated.

Apply the moisturizers with gentle, upward and outward motions. Remind yourself that you are creating a love affair with your face. Begin with your forehead, gently stroke upwards into the hairline using only your fingertips. Move to the upper cheek area, stroking lightly outwards, then move to the mouth area, smoothing upward and outward. These motions caress the face while allowing no stressful movements to aggravate the skin on the face, neck or chest.

Always apply the moisturizers using upward, outward strokes away from the mouth. The very act of stroking and massaging these potent "hydroscopic" materials promotes their function of attracting and binding moisture deep within your skin.

Apply the moisturizers to your upper chest, neck and back of the neck areas, even the back of your hands, stroking gently. The upper chest needs added moisture every day and applying the moisturizers will maintain that velvety feeling all day and night. Remember, the upper chest is prone to wrinkling from sun exposure and sleeping positions. All products that are used on your face and your neck need to be applied to the upper chest area and the back of your neck as well.

Allow the Day Cream to sit on your skin for a few minutes before applying foundation so that "rolling" does not occur. Rolling takes place if you apply your foundation without allowing the cream to penetrate the skin. This means that your foundation, your day cream and any other treatment you have applied will roll off if insufficient time has elapsed between applications. You do not want that to happen. I usually curl my eyelashes or help myself to a cup of coffee after applying the Day Cream so that it has time to penetrate.

Cynthia's Nighttime Regimen for the Face

The nighttime regime is devoted to tissue regeneration. It is during sleep that your body and skin experience rejuvenation.

1. Facial Magic detergent free Cleanser
2. Vitamin C Serum
3. Facial Magic Eye Treatment
4. Retinol. Retinol is a potent age-defying treatment. Retinol, the most active form of Vitamin A, has been proven to be exceptionally effective in reducing the visible signs of aging. The Retinol I use is advanced technology that delivers the purest form of bio-available Retinol deep within the skin. Your skin will feel firmer as it works to visibly reduce discoloration, fine lines and wrinkles. Allow the Retinol to penetrate your skin before applying your Night Cream. This is available at www.cynthiarowland.com.
5. Facial Magic Overnight Sensation. Apply just like you would the Facial Magic Daytime Skin Nutrition

"I am alert and exhilarated about life."

Chapter Ten – Essential Oils vs. Pharmaceutical Drugs

I have recently been introduced to the power and healing benefits of essential oils for treating both common and complex human health challenges. Essential oils are highly potent aromatic liquids extracted from shrubs, flowers, trees, roots, bushes and seeds.

Ancient civilizations dating back to 4500 BC used essential oils in religious ceremonies and medical applications. You may recall that the Three Wise Men brought gold, Frankincense and Myrrh to commemorate the birth of Jesus. Frankincense and Myrrh are essential oils regarded as valuable as gold at the time.

I cannot recount the multitude of information on essential oils in this chapter. I have found that the most comprehensive guide to essential oils is D. Gary Young's "Essential Oils Pocket Reference" available at www.youngliving.com.
Essential oils are my first choice in treating unhealthy conditions. They never lose their potency or effectiveness. They have intelligence and were divinely provided us as powerful substances to alleviate sickness, maladies and disease.

With over 100 trillion cells working together to keep us healthy, it's refreshing to know that essential oils heal the body and the skin but drugs do not. Prescription medicines whether taken internally or applied topically always have side effects – essential oils work to communicate with the body.

Some months ago I interviewed David Stewart, PhD, author of "The Chemistry of Essential Oils Made Simple" on The Ageless Sisters Blog Talk Radio show, regarding Young Living Essential Oils. He had this to say, "Non-toxic natural organic substances are usually easily eliminated by the body when their usefulness has run their course. Up to a point, your body can even deal with and eliminate natural toxic substances. But when your body receives a synthetic substance, even one that may seem benign or inert (like plastic), your body does not know how to metabolize and eliminate it. If sent to the liver to break it down into disposable compounds, the liver says, "Hey. What is this? I don't know what to do with it. Here kidneys, you take it." Then the kidneys react saying, "Hey liver, don't send it to us. We don't know what it is either. Send it to the pancreas. Maybe it will have an enzyme that can deal with it." Then the pancreas objects, "Hey guys, what do you think you are doing? I don't want this stuff. Dump it in the blood or the lymph or try the spleen. Maybe the spleen can filter this thing out or something." Finally, the substance ends up in the long term waste holding area of the body (usually fat tissue, including the brain) where it can remain for years and even for a lifetime, perturbing normal body functions as long as it remains. That's why you can find traces of prescription drugs in your body taken in childhood, decades ago.

On the other hand, natural molecules, such as those found in essential oils, are easily metabolized by the body. In fact, your body was created to handle them. When an essential oil molecule finds the receptor sites it was designed to fit and conveys its information to the cell, or participates in other therapeutic functions, it then goes on its way to the liver and the kidneys and moves out of the body. Its benefits have been conveyed and its job is complete.

By contrast, the unnatural molecules of man-made drugs attach themselves to various tissues, disrupting normal function for years while the body tries to figure out what to do with them. Meanwhile, they wreak mischief with our bodily functions and even our minds."

Dr. Stewart goes on to say: "Drugs and oils work in opposite ways. Drugs toxify. Oils detoxify. Drugs clog and confuse receptor sites. Oils clean receptor sites.

Drugs depress the immune system. Oils strengthen the immune system. Antibiotics attack bacteria indiscriminately, killing both the good and the bad. Oils attack only the harmful bacteria, allowing our body's friendly flora to flourish.

Drugs are one-dimensional, programmed like robots to carry out certain actions in the body, whether the body can benefit from them or not. When body conditions change, drugs keep on doing what they were doing, even when their actions are no longer beneficial.

Essential oils are multi-dimensional, filled with homeostatic intelligence to restore the body to a state of healthy balance. When body conditions change, oils adapt, raising or lowering blood pressure as needed, stimulating or repressing enzyme activity as needed, energizing or relaxing as needed. Oils are smart. Drugs are dumb.

Drugs are designed to send misinformation to cells or block certain receptor sites in order to trick the body into giving up symptoms. But drugs never deal with the actual causes of disease. They aren't designed for that purpose. While they may give prompt relief for certain uncomfortable symptoms, because of their strange, unnatural design, they will always disrupt certain other bodily functions. Thus, you always have some side effects."

Essential oils can treat acne, dry skin, reduce wrinkles, balance oily skin, alleviate sensitive skin and even improve skin's elasticity.

What are the recommended essential oils for skin care? Lavender, Sacred Frankincense, Geranium, Rose, Patchouli, Sage and Myrrh are my recommendation. Just use a drop in your lotion and gently massage into the affected areas.

Prescription and illegal drugs can have an adverse affect in your body which then shows on your skin. We've seen meth faces, faces that look tired, sagging and mostly unhealthy. How is it that something prescribed could wreak havoc with your skin to make it look tired and unappealing? Even anti-depressants and pain pills can relax the facial muscles and make your face look saggy.

I get all of my essential oils from Young Living (http://www.youngliving.com) because the oils are of the highest quality and potency. Young Living is a network marketing organization. At this writing, I have not sponsored anyone into the organization. If you would like to join the Young Living organization, send me an email at cyntha@cynthiarowland.com. I would be honored to sponsor you.

"I am renewed in mind, body and spirit."

Chapter Eleven – Facial Exercises – What to Expect

Getting started with Facial Magic exercises is easy. The goal is to lift your sagging facial muscles, strengthen them and see the results quickly. The desire for a younger looking face is a lifetime commitment. The benefits of seeing a younger looking face for the rest of your life is a fantastic incentive to learn Facial Magic and maintain your results so that you always look younger than your years.

In the beginning: once a day, six days a week...

Each exercise is performed once a day for six consecutive days for at least fifteen weeks to ensure that each muscle group sufficiently benefits from the program. Initially, I exercised my face Monday through Saturday, taking Sunday off and I believe that is a good routine for you.

Each contraction is held for a Five Second Count, then Ten seconds, Ten seconds, and Ten seconds.

Each exercise requires thirty five seconds of contraction. The first movement is held for five seconds, and then three additional repetitions are performed and held for ten seconds each. Do not rush "the count." There is a Voice CD that counts the cadence for you included in the DVD Systems available at www.cynthiarowland.com.

In the beginning exercise once a day, six days in a row for best results.

A Mirror is a must...

The exercises require your full attention. You may either stand or sit in front of your mirror. Personally, I like to stand because it gives me the opportunity to tighten my stomach muscles as I breathe and concentrate. Your hand placement, your finger placement, and your facial posture all contribute to your success. *Your results are achieved when you are in front of your mirror.*

By yourself. Undisturbed. Always examine the placement of your fingers to make certain you are not squinting or wrinkling any area of your face before performing your exercises. Study the photos and illustrations for the correct positioning of your fingers and hands. Even if you are familiar with the movements, it is a good idea to re-check your positioning from time to time.

Gloves are a must...

Gloves are required on some of the exercises. Wearing these white cotton gloves is crucial to your success. Facial Magic employs a special technique called "anchoring" that requires a thumb or finger placement inside your mouth. The gloves will allow you to anchor your muscles successfully. Keep your gloves clean by washing them frequently. Just lay them on a towel to dry rather than using your dryer. These gloves are available at www.cynthiarowland.com.

Anchoring is unique...

Anchoring a muscle creates a contraction in the muscle. A facial muscle is connected to a bone on only one end. The other end is connected to either another muscle or to tissue rather than a bone. This means that you must create the other anchor and you do this with either your forefingers or thumbs. This action produces the necessary resistance to insure a solid, sustainable contraction. Without the resistance ("anchoring technique") there is nothing for the muscle to work *against* that would produce the tension required to build and strengthen the muscle.

Learn two exercises a week...

Facial Magic introduces you to two new exercises per week. In Week One you learn the Upper Cheek and Upper Eye exercises. That is the extent of your first week's training. Two exercises only, a total of seventy seconds daily in front of your mirror. In Week Two you add two additional exercises, one for your Jowls, and one for your Pouches, so now you are exercising two minutes and twenty seconds each day. In Week Three the exercises address your Neck and Double Chin, which adds another minute or so to your daily routine.

> *Learn two exercises each week to look 10 -15 years younger in just 12 weeks. Take your beginning photo now. No smiling.*

Weeks Four and Five work your Upper Lip, Lower Eye, Vertical Forehead Lines and your Chin & Lower Lip. Week Six and Week Seven will introduce another Neck exercise, Horizontal Forehead Lines, another Lower Eye movement and the first Back of Cheeks exercise. Weeks Eight and Nine work on Crow's Feet, more Back of Cheeks for contour, the Bridge of the Nose and your Laugh Lines.

And so it goes for nine weeks. The slow introduction process is essential to your success with this program because specific muscles must be strengthened first to build that all important muscle foundation. As you become more familiar with the movements, you will move easily from one exercise to the next.

Added benefits...

From the beginning of your Facial Magic program, you will enjoy other benefits such as improved posture. As your neck muscles strengthen, you will notice that your face feels firmer, your skin looks healthier with a smoother texture, and the symptoms of muscle atrophy will be dramatically reduced.

Expect to see a difference...

In the very first week, you will notice subtle differences. You will see your upper eye area responding, and your cheek muscles will feel stronger. Most women say that definite changes are seen in the very first week. Whether you are thirty years old or eighty years young, you will love your results!

"I appreciate greater awareness in all areas of my life."

Chapter Thirteen – Workbook

A note from Cynthia:

Dear Friend:

I am delighted that you are beginning the Facial Magic program! It is with you in mind that I developed this multi-faceted regimen of facial exercises, special skin care and nutrition. The book and the workbook are designed to promote a toned, younger, more vibrant facial appearance in everyone! The Facial Magic process of rejuvenation has taken years to produce and I take great pride in sharing it with you.

This proven, safe and effective method of facial rehabilitation offers you a natural way to deal with sagging muscles.

In just a few weeks, you will see positive, lasting results. I would love to hear about your experiences with this program. Each of you has something unique and special to share so please email me at *cynthia@cynthiarowland.com* and send before and after photos. We're always looking for that next success story.

Please nurture yourself! Laced throughout the workbook, you will find "daily thoughts" and beauty tips to enhance your efforts toward self-improvement. Your healthy attention to your appearance will reflect in a positive image throughout all aspects of your life.

Enjoy your new face!
Best,
Cynthia

THE FACE:

A REFLECTION OF AGING, ATROPHY AND STRESS

Our faces give people their first impressions, an imprint that can be significant throughout our lives.

Our faces can shine forth and reflect our attention to health and vigor of body, mind and spirit or the face can blatantly shout that we are wearing the ravages of stress, gravity and facial tissue atrophy. Unfortunately, we cannot disguise this challenge with a new hairdo, make-up or special creams.

How and when did the facial drooping and sagging develop? What can we do to stop it? How can we correct unwanted jowls, double chins or droopy upper eyes? Why must the aging process represent a loss in facial muscular tone when common practice in other areas of physical fitness shows that significant improvements can be achieved with exercise?

THE SOLUTION:

THE FACIAL MAGIC PROGRAM

Remember: Consult your physician before starting the Facial Magic exercise program or any other exercise program.

WORKBOOK FEATURES & BENEFITS

The Facial Magic System is a facial exercise program designed to strengthen and contour the underlying muscles of your face and neck.

You will enhance your appearance and enjoy greater confidence.

THE BENEFITS INCLUDE:

Strengthened facial muscles

Improved skin tone

Improvements seen almost immediately

Easy to learn method

Safe for men and women over the age of 25

Complete initial toning in just 12 weeks

Quick: only minutes of exercise per day

Lifted youthful appearance

Greater confidence and satisfaction

Better posture

FACIAL MAGIC®

HOW THE FACIAL MAGIC PROGRAM WORKS

THE FACIAL EXERCISE PROCESS

The Facial Magic program uses isometric contractions to produce smoother skin and a healthier glow from increased oxygen and blood supply to the facial area. Muscles are strengthened to create a toned, contoured, lifted appearance.

Facial Magic exercises teach how to create a contraction by using your fingers to anchor the muscles, which allows them to shorten over time with consistent exercise. Our facial muscles are much smaller than most muscles so they respond quickly to exercise. Most muscles in the face are attached to the skin. Facial skin and the hidden muscles underneath must be handled delicately to achieve positive results.

You will learn two exercises per week. Every ensuing week, you will add another two movements so that at the end of the initial nine-week program, you will be performing eighteen exercises.

Your mind and your muscles will work together to produce your desired results.

Wearing Facial Magic special exercise gloves are required and will enhance your performance.

LET THE MAGIC BEGIN ...

Aging in your face begins with your muscles losing their tone due to the lessened production of collagen and elastin. Atrophy results. We see the effects of this in other parts of our bodies, too. Our thighs become less defined, our waists thicken and our derriere has a mind of it's own. We can cover and camouflage our body with long jackets, long skirts, turtlenecks, etc., but our faces are "out there". They are our calling cards, our power suits.

The Facial Magic exercise program addresses all areas of the face and neck. Our facial muscles are different. They weave over and under other muscle groups and then connect only one end to bone. When the slackening of the muscle begins, it often sags or "pools" into another muscle grouping, creating a line or a *wrinkle* in our face. The longer that muscle sags and pushes into another muscle or muscle group, the line or wrinkle becomes more permanent. Facial Magic will strengthen your muscles and help them to become more youthfully aligned. Your face will benefit from this unique toning process and you will look radiant and fresh.

As the muscles rehabilitate, wrinkling on your face will become less apparent as "lifting" occurs. If you have been worried about jowls, pouches, sagging cheeks, a tired eye area, this workbook combined with the exercises will definitely change all that.

Facial Magic addresses fifteen regions of the face and neck with eighteen exercises that you will initially complete in fifteen weeks. For the first nine weeks you will learn two exercises per week. It is recommended that you perform each exercise every day for six consecutive days and then enjoy one day of rest.

There are many benefits to using Facial Magic: radiant skin, a toned face, better posture and a positive self image are but a few of the perks of Facial Magic. As you move through the workbook, I want to offer you the best advice possible so that you are successful with the program and delighted with your results.

The success of this program is in your hands, literally. You are about to embark on a specialized training program that puts you in charge of your face.

OBSERVATIONS

I would like you to indicate the advantages you hope to achieve with a more youthful appearance. This is your workbook to use everyday, as you begin the adventure of creating a love affair with your face.

○ **Greater confidence**	○ **Greater Desirability**	○ **Meet People Easier**
○ **Meet More People**	○ **More Activity Choices**	○ **Look Healthier**
○ **Avoid Rejection**	○ **More Calm/Less Stress**	○ **Look More Natural**
○ **Use Less Make-up**	○ **Look More Successful**	○ **Be More Admired**
○ **Income Potential**	○ **Better Job Prospects**	○ **Less Work Hours**
○ **Appear Less Tired**	○ **Avoid Discrimination**	○ **Security**
○ **More Respect**	○ **Less Self Conscious**	○ **More Job Freedom**
○ **More Authority**	○ **Better Work Relations**	○ **Look More Intelligent**
○ **Self Importance**	○ **Love Relations Improved**	○ **Attract Suitable Mate**
	○ **Appear More Capable**	

Just check any of the boxes you feel applies to you. No one needs to know the answers but you. Be honest in how you feel right now about your facial appearance. Close your eyes and visualize that face you had ten to twenty years ago. Maybe you can find a photo that best represents you. It doesn't matter if the photo is twenty years old. Place it in your workout area so that you can see yourself often.

Muscles have memory and your brain is very powerful, so the combination of seeing the photo daily helps refresh the memory of yourself.

Look at your face in the mirror. What areas would you most like to improve?

Here is a checklist for you to indicate the areas in which you would welcome change:

- Upper Cheeks
- Lower Eye
- Upper Eyes
- Jowls
- Pouches Below Mouth Corners
- Upper Lip
- Chin and Lower Lip
- Forehead

- Turkey Neck
- Vertical Forehead Lines
- Horizontal Forehead Lines
- Bridge of Nose
- Back of Cheeks & Temple
- Lower Cheeks & Mouth Corners
- Crows Feet
- Neck & Double Chin

Our facial muscles know how they are supposed to look and we are going to retrain them. Just how is it that they sag? As we age, the muscle tissue begins to lose tone because of lack of use. The reason is that our facial muscles are very seldom tensed or contracted. That is what happens. When you smile, laugh, or sing, you use your muscles but that motion does not create a tensing motion or a contraction. Try it. Can you tense your facial muscles?

The facial muscles are not connected to bone in the same manner as our skeletal muscles, i.e., bone, hinge, bone with muscles in between, connected to another hinge/bone combination. Your skeletal muscles work by tightening and creating tension. A good example of this is when you pick up a barbell. The muscles in your arm immediately tense and contract as the barbell is lifted. Your muscles flex and tense because the muscles are anchored to your bones and joints. The Facial Magic movements employ the use of your fingers to act as "anchors," because without anchoring (resistance), your muscles cannot tense or contract. Some of the Facial Magic exercises require either a thumb or finger *inside* the mouth to grasp the end of a muscle. Each exercise is thoroughly explained so that you can easily understand and perform the movements.

YOUR PERSONAL OBSERVATIONS

This is your personal journal for facial rejuvenation.

Please take the time to fill out this questionnaire. You are the only one who will see it so just tell it like it is.

Date _Dec 9, 2021_

Job description _retired_

Is your job stressful? _____ How? _____

Is there another profession you would prefer? _____
If so, describe_____

What do you do for relaxation? _read, travel, thrift, cook_

How often do you exercise? _daily for stomach_

What type of exercise suits you best? _isometric_

List the vitamins you take: _D3, C, Biotin, Mag & Zinc_

Do you have health problems or concerns? _allergies (dust mites)_

List all surgeries over the past five years: _none_

FACIAL MAGIC®

Are you under the care of a physician? _yes_

Describe ___Dr. Ashley Trexler___

___

List all the medications you take: _zyrtec, flonase (allergies) zetia (cholesterol)_
HCT (40 pill) baby aspirin + supplements

Are you in good health? _yes_ Neck injuries? _no_ Smoke? _no_

Do you wear foundation daily? _yes_ Blush? _yes_ Mascara? _yes_ Lipstick? _yes_

Do you wash your face nightly? _yes_

Do you moisturize your face nightly? _yes_

Do you have regular facials? _no_ Any allergies to skin products? _no_

Shampoo frequency: _3X a wk_ Beauty Salon frequency: _none_

Do you eat red meat? _yes_ How many times per week? _1 or 2_

Current weight _142_ Ideal weight _135_ Are you on a diet? _yes (atkins)_

Do you have sun-damaged skin due to overexposure to sunlight or tanning lamps and beds? _yes_

Do you have or have you been treated for TMJ? _no_

Describe your skin condition: _presently 75 yrs. old - everything_
is popping up now - brown spots, crusty skin
crepey

Any other observations? _have started gua sha & other in facial exercise_
and noticed a difference, hence, bought this book

Facial Magic is a method that concentrates solely on you. It requires you to be undisturbed - in front of a mirror, beginning the creation of a love affair with yourself. There is no one more important than you and Facial Magic is a stepping-stone for your personal growth.

FACIAL MUSCLE ATROPHY: WHAT DOES IT MEAN?

Body tissues need nourishment and exercise to function at peak efficiency and achieve optimal health and appearance.

Atrophy is simply defined as "disuse of your muscles". When this condition occurs, you may experience any of the following symptoms and conditions:

• Puffiness due to edema, which is an excessive accumulation of fluid in your tissues.

• Hollowness in your upper cheek area

• Loss of elasticity and tone in the skin

• Shifts in muscle tissue that drags your skin in ways that either reveal your age or accentuate it

• Muscle elongation and sagging of both muscle and skin

Facial Magic addresses the underlying problem of muscle atrophy. Why is Facial Magic so unique? Because it works!

WORKBOOK TOOLS FOR SUCCESS

The Facial Magic System provides the following tools for success:
• A comprehensive demonstration of all the exercises
• A comprehensive workbook
• An exercise schedule to chart your progress
• A personal journal to record before and after photos along with your observations to monitor your results
• Recommendations for a comprehensive approach to managed skin care
• Daily affirmations to reinforce your positive approach to growth, self-esteem and self-enrichment.

SUCCESS REGIMEN - "PRACTICE MAKES PERFECT"
EXERCISE TIME, RELAXATION & ENVIRONMENT

Choose a time of day for performing your exercises when you are most likely to be relaxed and when you do not feel rushed. Select an atmosphere where you will not be disturbed so that you can concentrate on the program and you.

CONSISTENCTY & REST

All exercises should be performed six (6) consecutive days a week. Exercise only once a day. On the seventh day, do not perform any exercises as this is a day of rest for your face.

Keep your Progress Chart up to date. Note any days that you miss with a "-".

FACIAL MAGIC®

CLEANLINESS (HYGIENE)

Prepare for the exercise program by making certain that your face is absolutely clean. If you are prone to extremely dry skin, you may lightly moisturize your face; however, your grip and contractions will be more effective if your face is thoroughly clean.

OBSERVATION

Always perform your exercises in front of a mirror. This is necessary so you can examine your face. Make certain that you are not squinting or wrinkling any area of your face while performing the exercise movements.

TECHNIQUE & POSITIONING

Learn the exact positioning of your hands by carefully studying the photos and reading the accompanying text that fully describes each movement.

• Positioning is your key to success
• Slow and careful movements are best! They promote your desired results!
• Gradually tense your muscles with steady, accurate movements as opposed to quick, jerky movements. Faster results are achieved from slower exercise movements. The same principles apply to facial exercises as to muscular exercises for other parts of your body.

It is imperative that you clear your mind so that you can focus on the particular muscle group that is being exercised at a given time. Refer frequently to the detailed descriptions in this workbook, to the photo references in the Facial Magic book, or demonstrations on the video tape.

REMINDER: BREATHE!

Between each repetition, remove your hands from your face and take a deep breath through your nose. Exhale through your nose. Your muscles need the extra oxygen! Tighten your abdominal muscles as you exhale. You'll be pleasantly surprised with your results.

Do not wait longer than 10-15 seconds before resuming the remaining sets of exercise.

MANNERISMS AND FACIAL POSTURE

Frowning, squinting, pursing your lips and other contortions of your face will have a definite effect over time. Learn to be conscious of these mannerisms. You can easily relax your face with a gentle touch by your ringer finger. For instance, when you feel a frown developing between your eyebrows, gently touch the area with your ring finger until you feel the frown relax.

Most vertical lines require special attention at night. During the course of your program, place a small piece of office tape over your frown lines before retiring. Believe it or not, the tape will not allow you to frown in your sleep!

"I ENJOY MY LIFE! I SMILE OFTEN!"

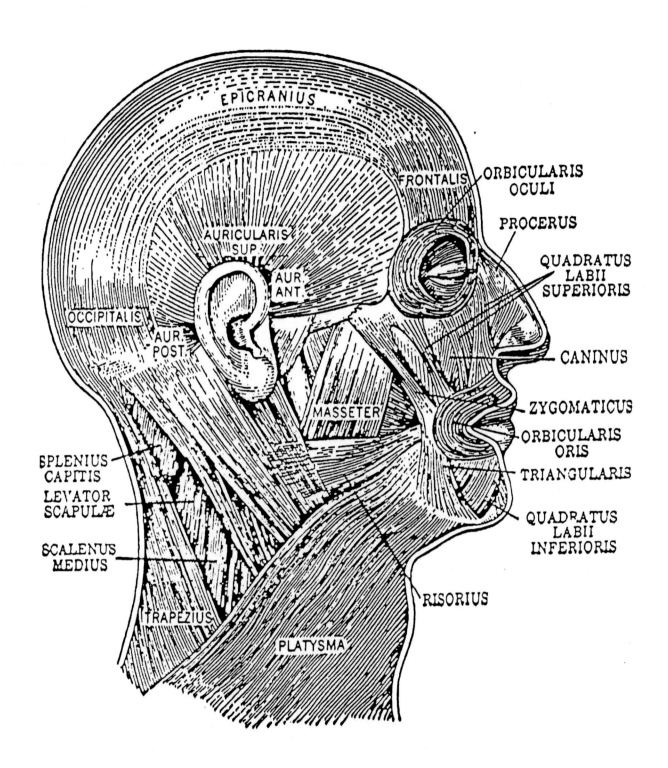

EPICRANIUS

FRONTALIS

ORBICULARIS
OCULI

PROCERUS

QUADRATUS
LABII
SUPERIORIS

CANINUS

ZYGOMATICUS

ORBICULARIS
ORIS

TRIANGULARIS

QUADRATUS
LABII
INFERIORIS

RISORIUS

AURICULARIS
SUP.

AUR.
ANT.

OCCIPITALIS

AUR.
POST.

MASSETER

SPLENIUS
CAPITIS

LEVATOR
SCAPULÆ

SCALENUS
MEDIUS

TRAPEZIUS

PLATYSMA

PERSONAL CHART
Weeks 1-4

(handwritten: 1/6/21)

Weeks:			1							2							3							4						
PLAN SEQUENCE		M	T	W	T	F	S	S	M	T	W	T	F	S	S	M	T	W	T	F	S	S	M	T	W	T	F	S	S
1	UPPER CHEEKS				✓	✓	✓	✓	✓	✓	✓	✓	✓	✓															
2	UPPER EYES				✓	✓	✓	✓	✓	✓	✓	✓	✓	✓															
3	JOWLS								✓	✓	✓	✓	✓	✓															
4	POUCHES								✓	✓	✓	✓	✓	✓															
5	NECK & DOUBLE CHIN																												
6	NECK & DOUBLE CHIN II																												
7	UPPER LIP																												
8	LOWER EYE																												
9	FOREHEAD LINES: VERTICAL																												
10	CHIN & LOWER LIP																												
11	FOREHEAD LINES: HORIZONTAL																												
12	NECK: TURKEY NECK																												
13	LOWER EYE II																												
14	BACK OF CHEEKS & TEMPLES																												
15	BACK OF CHEEKS II																												
16	CROWS FEET																												
17	BRIDGE OF NOSE																												
18	LAUGH LINES																												

EXERCISES

CHART INSTRUCTIONS: Chart your progress every day of your program. Perform the exercises in the order shown by the chart. This is correlated with the sequence shown in the book and the DVD.

FACIAL MAGIC®

PERSONAL CHART
Weeks 5-8

Weeks:		5							6							7							8						
PLAN SEQUENCE		M	T	W	T	F	S	S	M	T	W	T	F	S	S	M	T	W	T	F	S	S	M	T	W	T	F	S	S
1	UPPER CHEEKS																												
2	UPPER EYES																												
3	JOWLS																												
4	POUCHES																												
5	NECK & DOUBLE CHIN																												
6	NECK & DOUBLE CHIN II																												
7	UPPER LIP																												
8	LOWER EYE																												
9	FOREHEAD LINES: VERTICAL																												
10	CHIN & LOWER LIP																												
11	FOREHEAD LINES: HORIZONTAL																												
12	NECK: TURKEY NECK																												
13	LOWER EYE II																												
14	BACK OF CHEEKS & TEMPLES																												
15	BACK OF CHEEKS II																												
16	CROWS FEET																												
17	BRIDGE OF NOSE																												
18	LAUGH LINES																												

EXERCISES

After performing each set of exercises, check the appropriate box that coincides with the day of the week. If you skip a day, note that with a minus (-).

PERSONAL CHART
Weeks 9-12

Started

	Weeks:	9							10							11							12						
	PLAN SEQUENCE	M	T	W	T	F	S	S	M	T	W	T	F	S	S	M	T	W	T	F	S	S	M	T	W	T	F	S	S
1	UPPER CHEEKS				✓																								
2	UPPER EYES				✓																								
3	JOWLS																												
4	POUCHES																												
5	NECK & DOUBLE CHIN																												
6	NECK & DOUBLE CHIN II																												
7	UPPER LIP																												
8	LOWER EYE																												
9	FOREHEAD LINES: VERTICAL																												
10	CHIN & LOWER LIP																												
11	FOREHEAD LINES: HORIZONTAL																												
12	NECK: TURKEY NECK																												
13	LOWER EYE II																												
14	BACK OF CHEEKS & TEMPLES																												
15	BACK OF CHEEKS II																												
16	CROWS FEET																												
17	BRIDGE OF NOSE																												
18	LAUGH LINES																												

EXERCISES

Remember to take photos every three weeks of your Facial Magic training. Taking periodic photos allows you to better monitor your progress.

FACIAL MAGIC®

PERSONAL CHART
Weeks 13-16

Weeks:		13							14							15							16						
PLAN SEQUENCE		M	T	W	T	F	S	S	M	T	W	T	F	S	S	M	T	W	T	F	S	S	M	T	W	T	F	S	S
1	UPPER CHEEKS																												
2	UPPER EYES																												
3	JOWLS																												
4	POUCHES																												
5	NECK & DOUBLE CHIN																												
6	NECK & DOUBLE CHIN II																												
7	UPPER LIP																												
8	LOWER EYE																												
9	FOREHEAD LINES: VERTICAL																												
10	CHIN & LOWER LIP																												
11	FOREHEAD LINES: HORIZONTAL																												
12	NECK: TURKEY NECK																												
13	LOWER EYE II																												
14	BACK OF CHEEKS & TEMPLES																												
15	BACK OF CHEEKS II																												
16	CROWS FEET																												
17	BRIDGE OF NOSE																												
18	LAUGH LINES																												

EXERCISES

How Your Face Will Age Without Facial Magic

Mid 20's to mid 30's

- Frown lines begin to form between the brows.

Mid 30's to mid 40's

- Upper eyelids begin to gradually fall and hood the eye.
- Puffiness under the eye becomes apparent.
- Fine wrinkling shows around the eyes.
- The frown lines between the brows deepen.
- Lips begin to develop wrinkles and lose fullness.
- Folds and creases develop between nose and mouth.

Mid 40's to mid 50's

- Upper eyelids begin to gradually fall and hood the eye.
- Puffiness under the eye becomes apparent.
- Fine wrinkling shows around the eyes.
- The frown lines between the brows deepen.
- Lips begin to develop wrinkles and lose fullness.
- Folds and creases develop between nose and mouth.

Age 60 & over

- More of all of the above including more wrinkles and creases.

Chapter Fourteen – Week One Exercises

The zygomaticus muscle group (cheek muscle) covers our cheekbones; the levator labii superioris (cheek muscle) sits just behind the zygomaticus minor while the zygmaticus major connects to the orbicularis occuli (eye muscle).

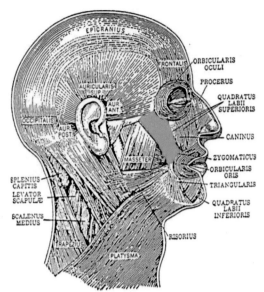

When atrophy begins, the muscles over your cheekbone elongate and "pool" (droop) into other muscles or muscle groups contributing to the fold or line that usually develops in this area. The almost imperceptible motion makes your skin sag over time. To counteract the pull of gravity, you need to elevate the muscles, awakening them, and creating a better blood supply to your cheek area by retraining and reshaping them so that they provide better support to your skin.

Put on your gloves. Make certain the gloves fit snugly over your fingertips and thumbs. Stand or sit in front of a mirror. Breathe in deeply through your nose and exhale through your nose.

1. Insert your thumbs vertically into your mouth between your upper lip and upper teeth.

2. Position your thumbs under the line or just outside of the line that appears from your nose to the corners of your mouth.

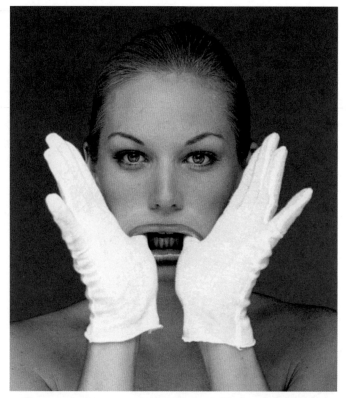

3. Nestle your index fingers horizontally, (first and second knuckles) under your cheekbones, on both sides of your nose and compress your thumbs and fingers gently together.

4. Gently pull straight down to fully extend the muscle, and hold. Keep your upper lip straight and drop your jaw slightly so that your mouth is open.

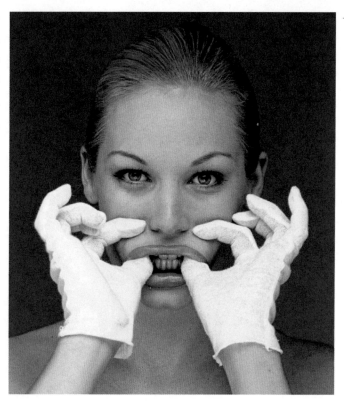

5. Now smile broadly to contract your upper cheek muscles. Hold the first contraction for five (5) seconds. Remember to keep your eye area relaxed, using only your cheek muscles. No squinting!

6. Remove your hands from your face.

7. Breathe in deeply through your nose and exhale through your nose.

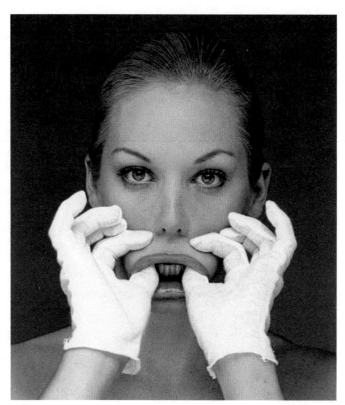

8. Repeat the three remaining sets, holding the contractions for ten (10) seconds each, remembering to count them out as one thousand one, one thousand two, one thousand three, etc.

9. Breathe in deeply through your nose and exhale through your nose.

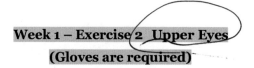

Week 1 – Exercise 2 Upper Eyes
(Gloves are required)

The frontalis muscle (forehead muscle) runs *vertically* over the forehead. You use it every time you lift your eyebrows. When this muscle begins to lose its tone, the frontalis begins to "pool" into the orbicularis oculi (the circular muscle that totally surrounds the eye). That motion affects the levator palpebra superioris (the muscle in your upper eye area). The eyelid begins to look hooded and then "the tired look" sets in. This exercise will increase the distance between your eyebrows and eyelashes, giving you a more refreshed appearance. You will feel the difference immediately!

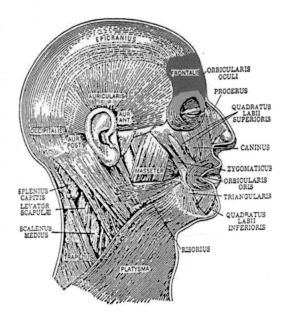

Sometimes you may be concerned that you are creating small horizontal lines above your eyebrows when you perform this exercise. The reason that lines may initially appear is because the forehead muscle has lost its tone. As you progress through the program these lines will begin to diminish, and by performing Exercise Eleven they will be greatly improved.

1. Relax your eyebrow area and then place the three middle fingers of each hand directly under your eyebrows.

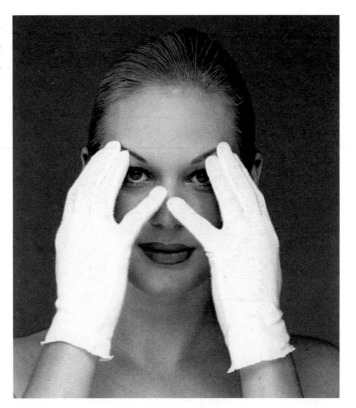

2. Drop the palms of your hands flat against your face.

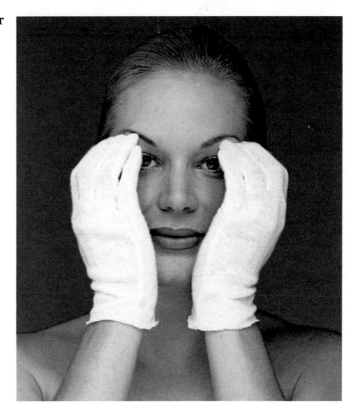

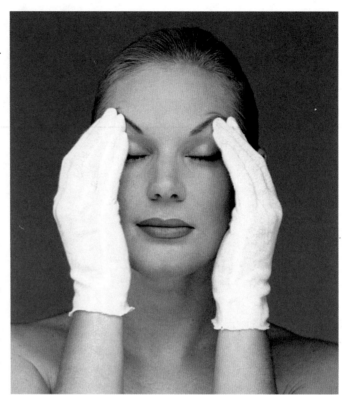

3. With the pads of your fingertips directly under your eyebrows, push your eyebrows upwards and slightly outwards.

4. Hold your eyebrows in this position with your eyes open.

5. Push your eyebrows down against your fingertips while holding your eyebrows high, and hold the contraction for five (5) seconds.

6. Remove your hands from your face.

7. Breathe in deeply through your nose, and exhale through your nose.

8. Repeat the three remaining sets holding the contractions for ten (10) seconds each. At the seventh second, close your eyes, keeping your eyebrows held high.

9. Remove your hands from your face. Breathe in deeply through your nose, and exhale through your nose.

Most likely your eyebrows responded immediately and you saw lifting. Perhaps you could see the difference for only a few seconds but it was there. This exercise will definitely lift your eyebrows, and the difference will become permanent over the next few weeks. Soon your friends will begin asking if you have changed your hair or your makeup routine. They will notice that something is different, but they will not be able to distinguish what the change is.

Special Eye Circle Exercise: Use your ring fingers, apply eye cream to your under eye areas using a dabbing motion.

Start by placing the tips of your ring fingers under your inner eyebrows and continue outward and then inward towards your nose until a full circle has been completed. Circle both eyes simultaneously, gently, with your ring fingers for one hundred times.

This easy exercise is performed very quickly. It is performed using a very gentle motion. No tugging, pulling, or stretching of the skin is allowed. It is an excellent way to increase the circulation to your eye areas, which helps to alleviate the appearance of dark circles under your eyes.

Week One Affirmations:

I am one with infinite life and wisdom.
I am energized!

Chapter Fifteen - Week Two Exercises

When the Zygomaticus muscles elongate, they push into our Orbicularis Oris muscle (the muscle that supports the area around the mouth). The loss of tone continues into the jaw area, creating the look of jowls and pouches. The next exercise will teach you how to firm this area.

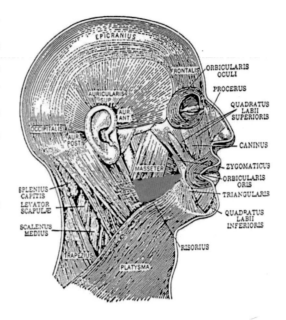

Complete the exercises on one side of the face before starting the other side.

1. While standing or sitting in front of your mirror, tilt your head back until you feel tension under your chin.

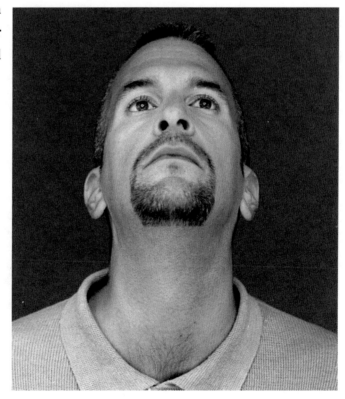

2. While keeping your head tilted, turn your head to the right and look over your shoulder, gently stretching your neck muscles.

3. Open your mouth slightly and jut out your bottom teeth and jaw. (This motion works the left side of your face)

4. Hold the contraction for five (5) seconds.

5. Relax your face; bring your head gently back to your original, level starting position. (Refrain from swinging your head around suddenly as you could strain your neck muscles.)

6. Breathe in deeply through your nose, and exhale through your nose.

7. Repeat the three remaining sets holding the contractions for ten (10) second each.

8. Breathe in deeply through your nose, and exhale through your nose.

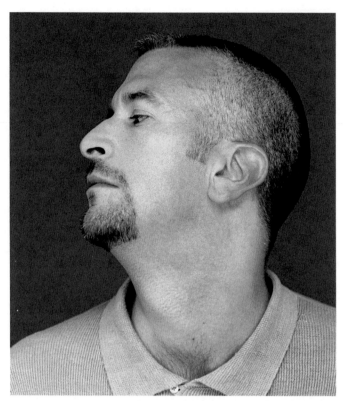

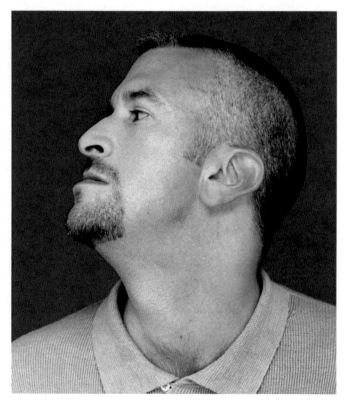

FACIAL MAGIC®

To exercise the right side of your face:

9. Tilt your head back until you feel the tension under your chin.

10. While keeping your head tilted, turn your head to the left and look over your shoulder.

11. Open your mouth slightly and jut out your bottom teeth and jaw.

12. Hold the first contraction for five (5) seconds then repeat the motion three times, holding the contractions for ten (10) seconds each.

13. Breathe in deeply though your nose and exhale through your nose.

You will feel the muscles in your neck elongate and the jaw muscles contract. This exercise allows a freer mobility when turning your head.

Week 2 – Exercise 4 Pouches
(Gloves are required)

Complete the exercises on one side of your face before starting the other side.

Pouches usually appear just below the corners of your mouth as little bulges. Pouches occur when the orbicularis oris (the circular muscle surrounding the mouth) has been compromised due to the additional weight of the zygomaticus pooling into the mouth region. This exercise will lift the entire cheek area and will help define your jaw line.

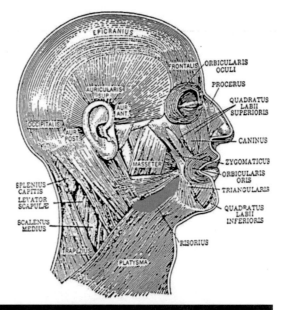

1. Insert your right thumb into the *left* side of your mouth at a downward angle just below the corner of your mouth and **compress** your mouth against your thumb. Keep your elbow elevated.

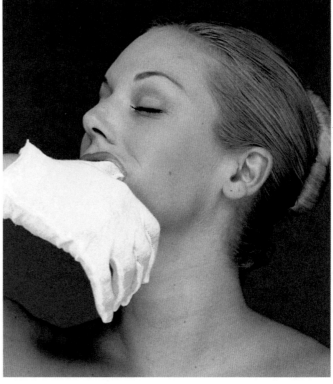

2. While compressing your mouth around your thumb, slightly push your thumb in an outward direction to create a contraction in your muscle. (If the area under your jaw is tense you will know that you have a contraction.) **Grip** the muscle between your curved index finger on the outside of your face and your thumb on the inside of your mouth.

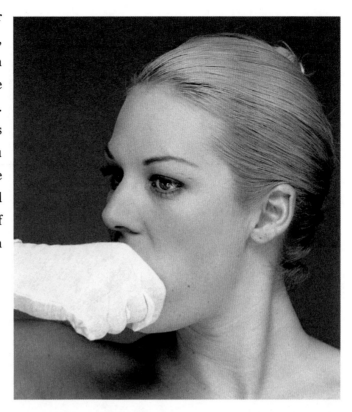

3. Support your right hand with your *left* hand. **Check in the mirror to make certain you are not creating wrinkling in any area of your face.**

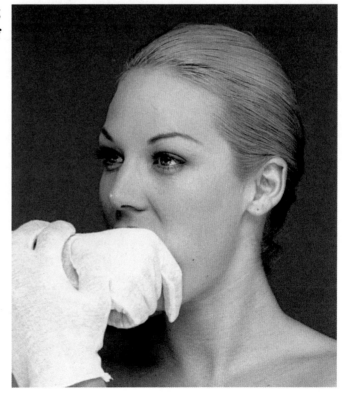

4. While you hold the muscle in place with your thumb, **contract** the gripped muscle toward your ear and hold for five (5) seconds. (At first you may not think you are making a contraction but indeed you are. In a few days, you will know that you are performing this particular exercise correctly.) **Do not pull or tug on your face in any way**.

5. Remove your hands.

6. Breathe in deeply through your nose and exhale through your nose.

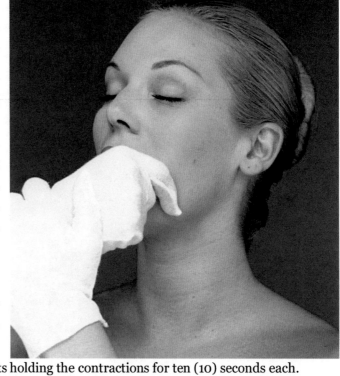

7. Repeat the three additional sets holding the contractions for ten (10) seconds each.

Now switch sides:

8. Insert your left thumb into the **right** side of your mouth at a downward angle just below the corner of your mouth and *compress* your mouth against your thumb. Keep your elbow elevated.

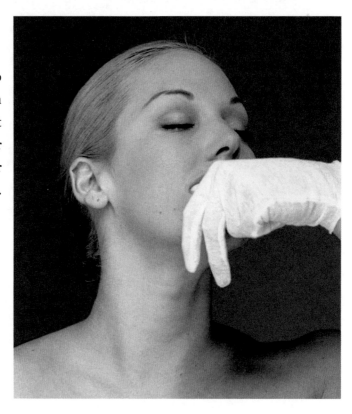

9. While compressing your mouth around your left thumb, push your thumb in an outward direction to create the contraction by tensing your mouth muscle. **Grip** the muscle between your curved index finger on the outside of your face and your thumb on the inside of your mouth.

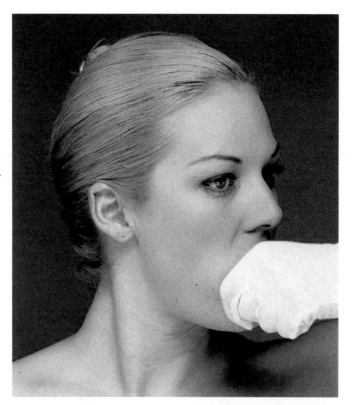

10. Support the grip with your right hand over the back of your left hand that is gripping the muscle. **Make certain you are not creating any wrinkling in any area of your face.**

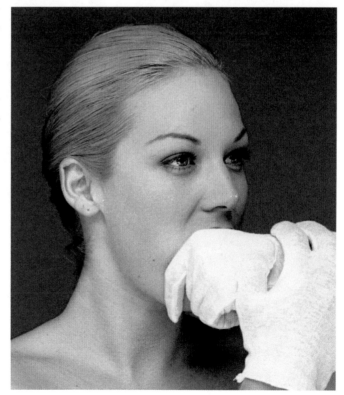

11. Do not pull or tug on your face, instead, simply hold the muscle in place with the pad of your thumb and **contract** the muscle back towards your ear. Hold the contraction for a count of five (5).

12. Remove your hands.

13. Breathe in deeply through your nose, and exhale through your nose.

14. Repeat the three additional sets holding the contractions for ten (10) seconds each.

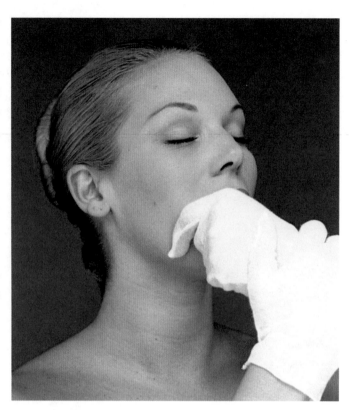

Week Two Affirmations:
I accept change in my life!
Divine order is at work!

Chapter Sixteen – Week Three Exercises

The broad, flat, thin Platysma muscle, (the neck muscle) is attached to the skin and extends between the front of your chest, (collarbone) and the lower edge of your jaw. It is just one of several important hidden structures that make up the bulk of your neck. When this muscle atrophies, fat can collect in the muscle tissue causing either a double chin or the dreaded "turkey neck". These neck exercises will tighten the muscles of your neck, helping your jaw line to become prominent again, creating a more youthful appearance.

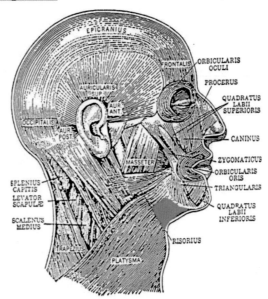

1. Lift your chin to create a taut line between your chin and the base of your neck. Keep your shoulders erect.
2. Clench your back teeth together.
3. Press the tip of your tongue against the inside of your lower gum line using your tongue as the anchor.

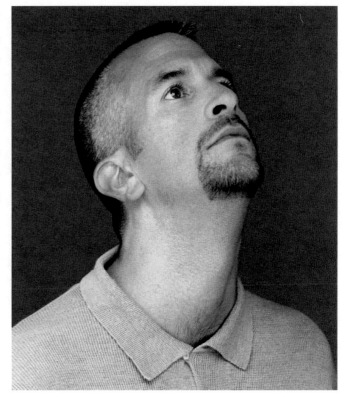

Tense your neck (This means that you are contracting the muscles of your neck) and hold for a count of five (5) seconds, one thousand one, one thousand two, one thousand three, etc.

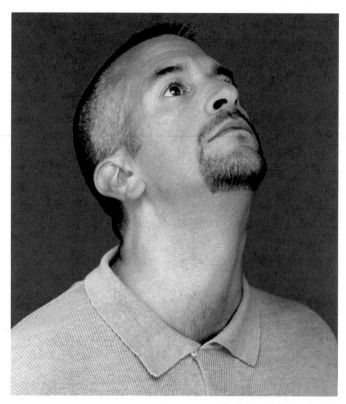

4. Relax your face and bring your head to its level position.
5. Breathe in deeply through your nose and exhale through your nose.
6. Repeat the three remaining sets holding the contractions for ten (10) seconds each.
7. Breathe in deeply through your nose and exhale through your nose.

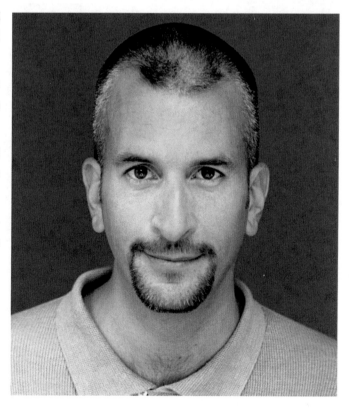

Week 3 – Exercise 6 Neck & Double Chin II
(No gloves required)

Exercise Six again addresses the broad Platysma muscle and extends the contraction throughout the neck.

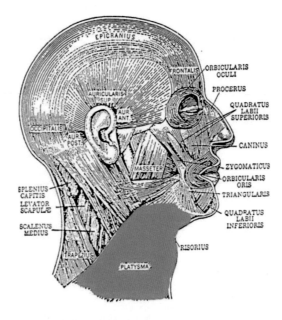

Lift your chin to create a taut line between your chin and the base of your neck. Keep your shoulders erect.

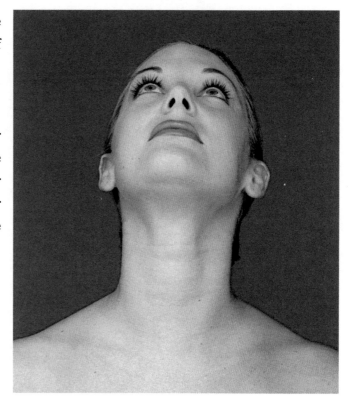

1. Press the surface of your tongue **firmly** against the roof of your mouth. (Your tongue acts as the anchor when you press it against the roof of your mouth.)

2. Allow your teeth and lips to part slightly.

3. Hold the contraction for five (5) seconds.

4. Relax your face and bring your head to its level position.

5. Breathe in deeply through your nose and exhale through your nose.

6. Repeat the remaining sets three times holding the contractions for ten (10) seconds each.

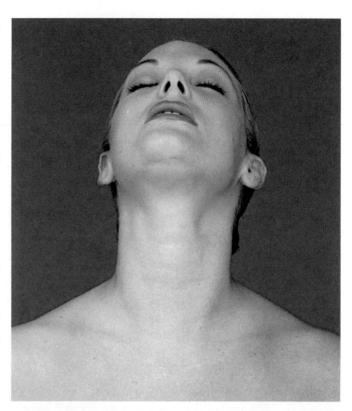

7. Breathe in deeply through your nose and exhale through your nose.

Week Three Affirmations:

I realize my personal power.

I exercise my power through my attitude, behavior, self-image, determination and commitment to life.

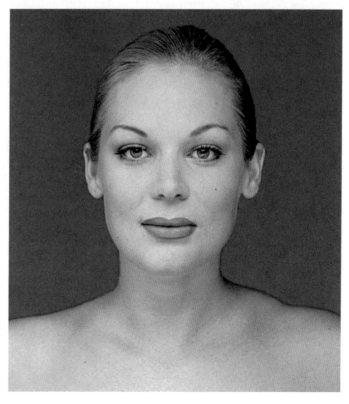

Chapter Seventeen – Week Four Exercises
Week 4 – Exercise 7 Upper Lip
(Gloves are required)

The orbicularis oris muscle is the chief muscle that forms a ring around your mouth. Like every muscle that is not specifically exercised, it becomes slack. As the slackness continues, lines develop above your lip. They may be tiny at first and then become apparent over time. Your lips may then look thinner and even withered. This exercise, along with the amazing Luscious Lips device (www.lippump.com) will keep your lips full. Your upper lip will be dramatically enhanced, your mouth will broaden and the corners of your mouth will turn upward.

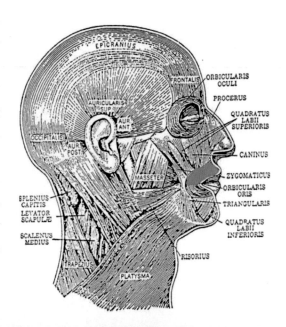

1. Put the heels of your hands together.

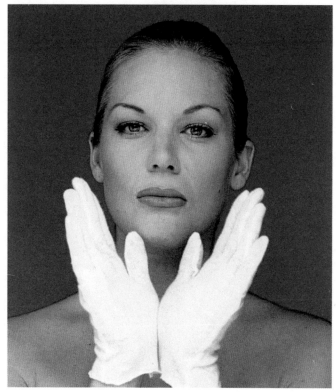

2. Insert your thumbs into your mouth under your upper lip in a "V" position and push your lip muscle outward without creating any lines around your mouth or lip area. Your entire upper lip surface should be smooth and oval in appearance.

3. Be aware of your facial posture. If you are accentuating the lines, reposition your thumbs until no lines are apparent. The goal for the upper lip is to be smooth and oval.

4. Lift your chin slightly.

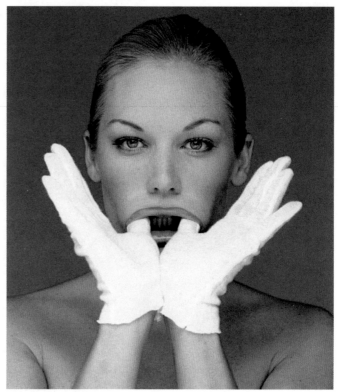

5. **Compress** your upper lip muscle against your thumbs. (Your thumbs act as anchors so when your muscle is contracted, the corners of your mouth will turn upward.)

6. Hold the contraction for a count of five (5) seconds

7. Remove your hands.

8. Breathe in deeply through your nose, and exhale through your nose.

9. Repeat the three remaining sets holding the contractions for ten (10) seconds each.

10. Breathe in deeply through your nose, exhale through your nose.

FACIAL MAGIC®

Week 4 – Exercise 8 Lower Eye
(No gloves required)

Strengthening your lower eye involves the orbicularis oculi muscle. This muscle surrounds your entire eye. Performing this exercise will strengthen your lower eye area.

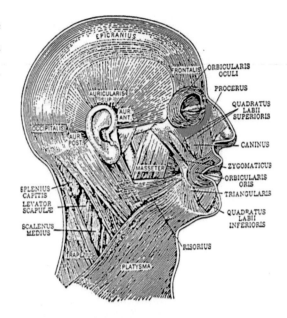

1. Start with your head level.
2. Turn your eyes upward ever so slightly while keeping your head level.

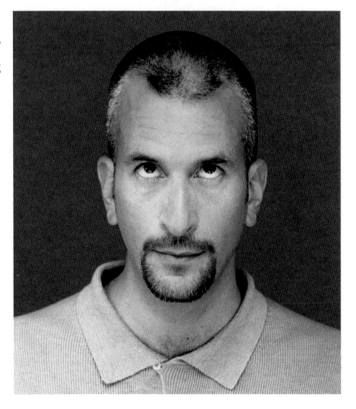

3. Begin to close your eyes from the bottom to the top lid and **glare** to tighten the lower eye muscle. (The movement is almost a squint but keep your eyes relaxed. You will feel like you are trying to force the muscle into the tear duct.) 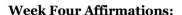 **Remember, DO NOT SQUINT OR WRINKLE YOUR FOREHEAD!** (With practice you will learn to glare without squinting or aggravating your crow's feet.)

4. Hold the glare for five (5) seconds.

5. Relax your eyes.

6. Breathe in deeply through your nose, and exhale through your nose.

7. Repeat the three remaining sets holding the contractions for ten (10) seconds each.

8. Breathe in deeply through your nose, and exhale through your nose.

Week Four Affirmations:

When we express gratitude for all we see, touch and feel, we find joy! I am joyful!

Chapter Eighteen – Week Five Exercises

Week 5 – Exercise 9 Vertical Forehead Lines
(Gloves are required)

The area between your eyebrows can be affected when we frown or concentrate. Sometimes one or even two lines can become apparent between your eyebrows. To soften the appearance of these lines, massage the area with your ring finger in a circular motion for a count of 100 little circles. Make certain that the area is kept moist with your hydrating moisturizer. Remember, if you feel a frown coming on, just touch the area between your eyebrows with your ring finger until the area is relaxed.

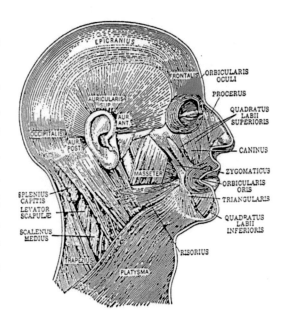

1. Hold your three middle fingers together and place them on each side of the vertical lines. Place your ring fingers under your inner eyebrows, positioned at their base. Place your index and middle fingers above your ring fingers on your forehead.

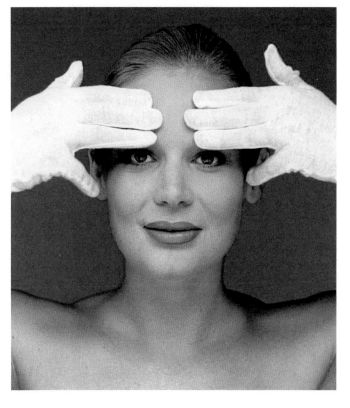

2. Gently pull your skin taut in an outward direction.
3. Raise the area by gently pushing upwards and hold.
4. While holding your forehead in the upward and outward position, bring your eyebrows together.
5. Hold for a count of five (5) seconds.
6. Remove your hands.
7. Breathe in deeply through your nose, and exhale through your nose.
8. Repeat the three remaining sets holding the contraction for ten (10) seconds each.

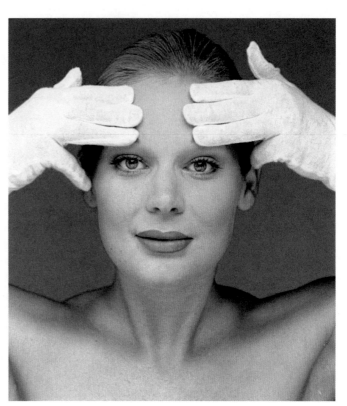

Week 5 – Exercise 10 Chin and Lower Lip
(No gloves required)

Sometimes when the face is losing its tone, you will see a faint line developing just under the lower lip. The following exercise not only rejuvenates the chin and lower lip, the effects radiate throughout the entire neck and jaw area.

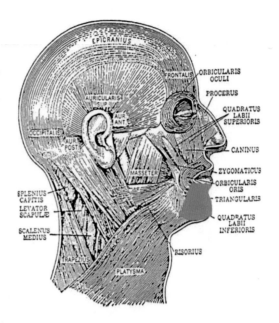

1. Hold your teeth and lips slightly apart.

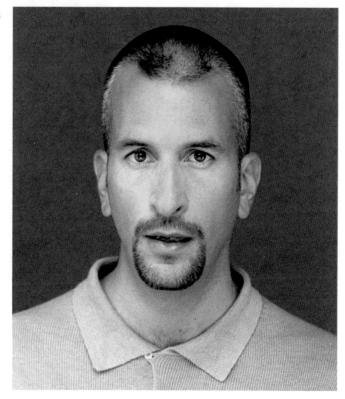

2. Curve your lower lip over your bottom teeth.

3. Force your lip and chin muscles in an outward direction by slightly tilting your chin upward.

4. Hold the count for five (5) seconds.

5. Bring your head level.

6. Relax your mouth.

7. Breathe in deeply through your nose, and exhale through your nose.

8. Repeat the three remaining sets holding the contraction for ten (10) seconds each.

Week Five Affirmations:

I am renewed and restored.

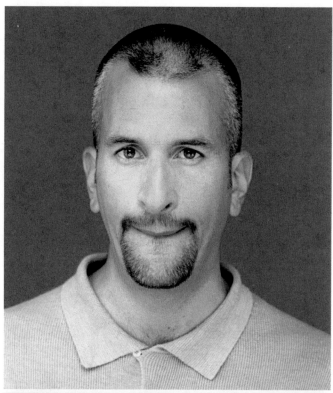

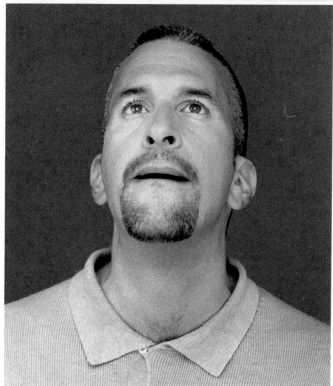

Chapter Nineteen – Week Six Exercises

Week 6 – Exercise 11 Horizontal Forehead lines
(Gloves are required)

The frontalis muscle affects the entire forehead. From the beginning of the exercise program, you have been strengthening this area, now it is time to contract the entire region. When your frontalis muscle loses its tone, the elongation of the muscle pushes into your eyebrows and also creates horizontal forehead lines.

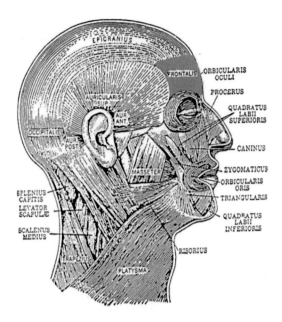

1. Place your thumbs above your temple area.
2. Apply pressure with your thumbs but do not pull the skin around your eye area.

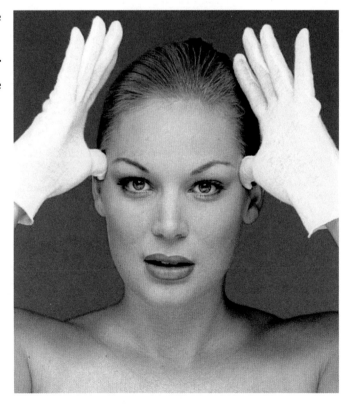

3. Position the three middle fingertips of your hands horizontally as close as possible to your hairline. Spread your fingers to cover the entire forehead area at your hairline.

4. With your fingertips, push your forehead up and hold.

5. Then using your forehead muscles, move your forehead in a downward movement against your fingertips. (Make certain you are not accentuating the vertical lines between your eyebrows. If you do see wrinkles reposition your fingertips until the area is unaffected.)

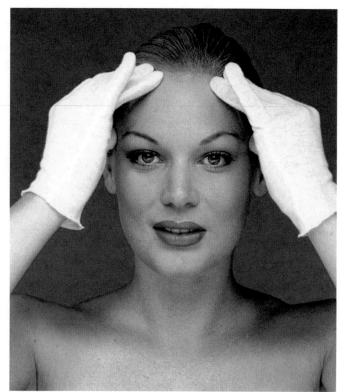

6. Hold the contraction for five (5) seconds.

7. Remove your hands.

8. Breathe in deeply in through your nose, and exhale through your nose.

9. Repeat the three remaining sets holding the contractions for ten (10) seconds each.

10. Breathe in deeply through your nose, and exhale through your nose.

Week 6 – Exercise 12 Neck
(No gloves required)

Your platysma muscle (the large, flat and broad neck muscle) has been strengthening since week two. Here is another movement to help tone the muscles of your neck. This exercise will be felt all the way to your collarbone and beyond. Some women say it can even help lift the bust line.

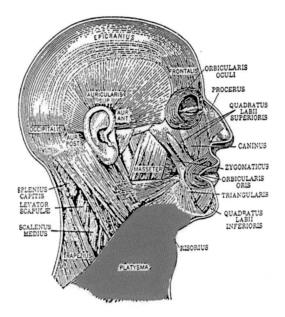

Tilt your head back to create a taut line from your chin to your clavicle.

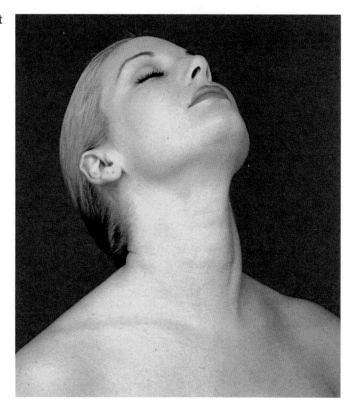

1. Extend your lower jaw and lip to accentuate the taut line.
2. Hold for a count of five (5) seconds.
3. Bring your head to its level position.
4. Breathe in deeply through your nose, and exhale through your nose.
5. Repeat the three remaining sets and hold the contractions for a count of ten (10) seconds each.
6. Breathe in deeply through your nose, and exhale through your nose.

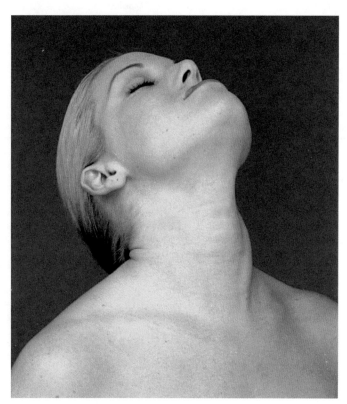

Week Six Affirmations:

I can accomplish any goal.

I complete one small task at a time, one day at a time.

Chapter Twenty – Week Seven Exercises

Week 7 – Exercise 13 Lower Eye II
(Gloves are required)

The lower eye muscle can be further improved by performing the following exercise.

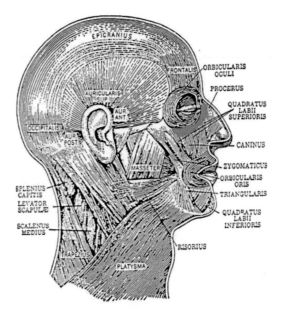

1. Lay the ring ringer of each hand under your lower lashes to cover as much of your under eye area as possible. Allow your fingers to slant slightly upwards toward the corners of your outer eyes.

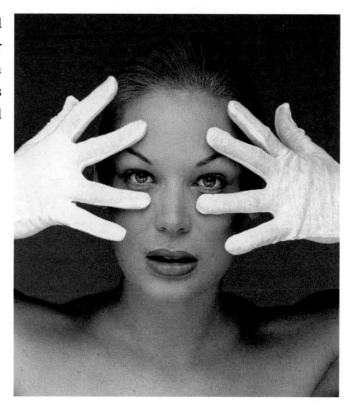

2. With gentle pressure and your ring fingers in position, look up slightly and **glare**. (You will feel the lower part of your eyeballs push against your fingers).

3. Keep your lead level and do not glare excessively.

4. Hold the first contraction for a count of five (5) seconds.

5. Remove your fingers.

6. Breathe in deeply through your nose, and exhale through your nose.

7. Repeat the three

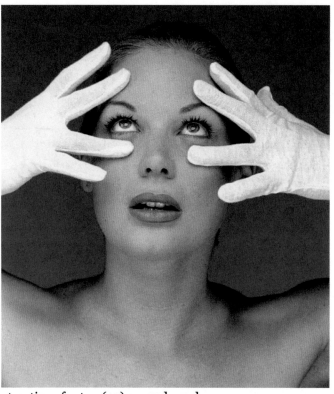

remaining sets holding the contractions for ten (10) seconds each.

8. Breathe in deeply through your nose, and exhale through your nose.

Week 7 – Exercise 14 Back of Cheeks
(No gloves required)

The following exercise helps strengthen the muscles near your ear and provides contour to your face. The movements encompass several muscles and muscle groups in the upper jaw area.

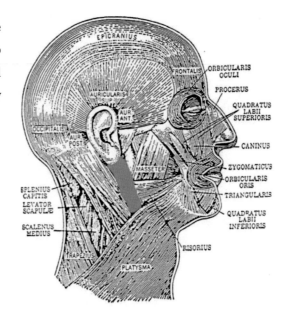

1. Wash your hands thoroughly with soapy water and rinse well.

2. With the backs of your hands touching, insert both index fingers into your mouth between your teeth and your cheeks.

3. Push your fingertips all the way back until you feel little "pads" at your fingertips.

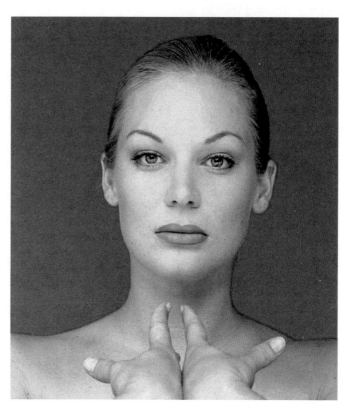

4. Do not pull the corners of your mouth or push out your cheeks.

5. Close your front teeth and **clench** your back teeth together.

6. While holding the "pads" (they are actually muscles) with your fingertips, flex the pads secured with your fingertips. Hold then release. (The flexing movement will show you that you are in the right position.)

7. Hold your fingertips against the pads for a count of five (5) seconds.

8. Remove your fingers.

9. Breathe in deeply through your nose, and exhale through your nose.

10. Repeat the three remaining sets holding the contractions for ten (10) seconds each.

11. Breathe in deeply through your nose, and exhale through your nose.

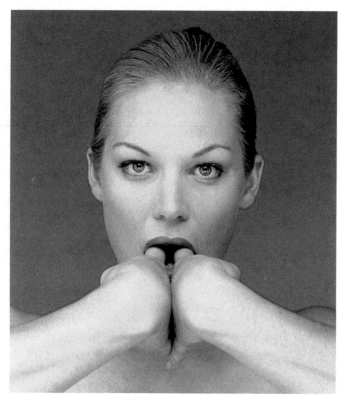

Week Seven Affirmations:
I love and accept others.
Only good is coming to me now.

Chapter Twenty-One – Week Eight Exercises

The following exercise is another movement that addresses the backs of your cheeks. The effect of this exercise creates a better contour to the sides of your face and can stop the hollowness that is sometimes seen in your upper cheek area.

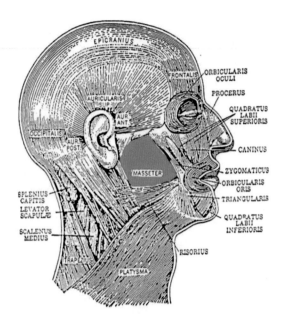

1. Place your forefinger and the middle finger of your dominant hand on your bottom teeth. Use one glove to cushion the area between your teeth and your fingertips.
2. Drop your jaw to extend the muscle and hold.

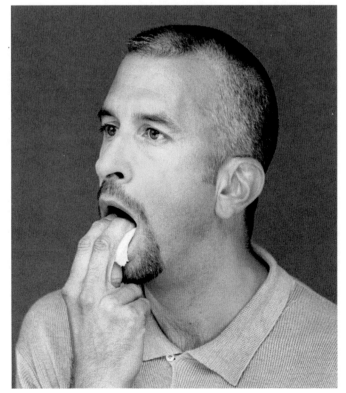

3. Contract your muscle by keeping your jaw in place while gently trying to close your mouth. (Use a very slow flexing motion so that you are creating tension in your upper jaw area.)

4. Hold the contraction for five (5) seconds.

5. Remove your fingers and your glove.

6. Breathe in deeply through your nose, and exhale through your nose.

7. Repeat the three remaining sets holding the contractions for ten (10) seconds each.

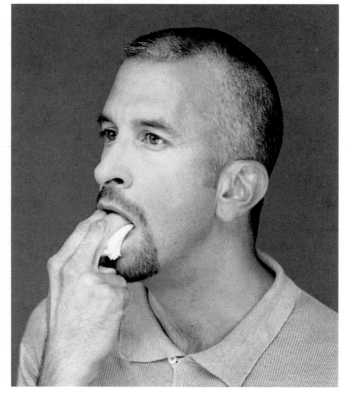

8. Breathe in deeply through your nose, and exhale through your nose.

Week 8 – Exercise 16 Crow's Feet
(Gloves are required)

Your very delicate eye area is prone to wrinkling and crinkling. The slackening of the frontalis muscle forces your forehead downwards into your eyebrows and that downward motion affects your skin. Your forehead has been rehabilitating since week one and you may have noticed that your crow's feet have diminished now that your underlying muscles are strengthening. The following exercise strengthens your entire eye area and primarily affects the area where crow's feet develop.

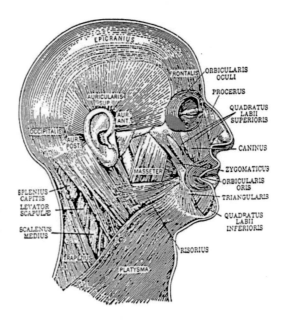

1.   Make a fist with both hands and extend your thumbs.
2.   Turn your hands upside down with your palms upward in a fist.

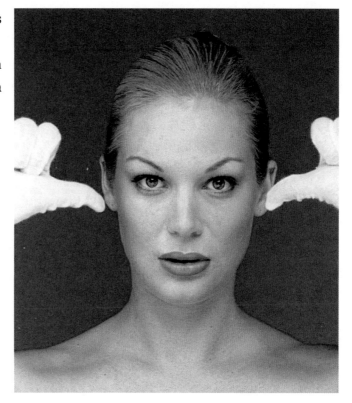

3. Press the pads of your thumbs against the bone next to the outside corners of your eyes.

4. Use gentle pressure against the bone but do not pull your skin.

5. Turn your eyes upward and allow your lower lids to close until your eyes begin to flutter.

6. Hold for a count of five (5) seconds

7. Remove your hands.

8. Breathe in deeply through your nose, and exhale through your nose

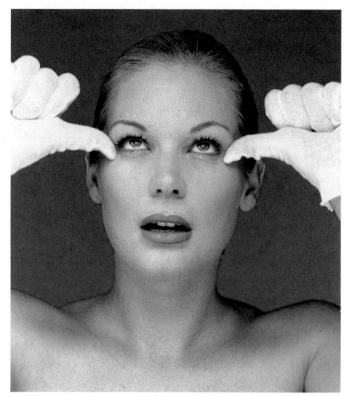

9. Repeat the three remaining sets holding the contractions for ten (10) seconds each.

10. Breathe in through your nose, and exhale through your nose.

Week Eight Affirmations:
My inner beauty is most valued by others.
I feel beautiful!

Chapter Twenty-Two – Week Nine Exercises

Week 9 – Exercise 17 Bridge of Nose
(Gloves are required)

Sometimes a little horizontal line can develop at the bridge of your nose. You have been conditioning your frontalis muscle for eight weeks and the following exercise is a refining exercise for this area of your face.

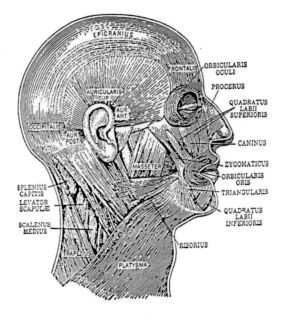

1. Place your middle finger of each hand below the horizontal line on the bridge of your nose. Make certain your fingertips are touching.

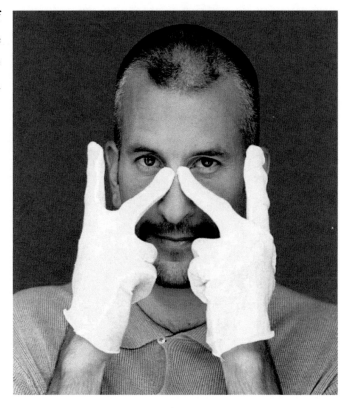

2. Gently extend the area by pulling the bridge area and hold. **Do not wrinkle your forehead**. (This takes practice and you will learn it quickly.)

3. Using your forehead muscle while your fingers anchor the skin, pull your forehead upward and hold for a count of five (5).

4. Remove your hands.

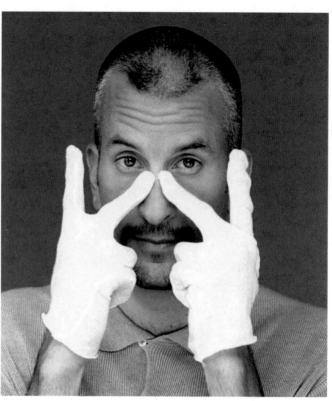

5. Breathe in deeply through your nose, and exhale through your nose.

6. Repeat the three remaining sets, holding the contractions for ten (10) seconds each.

7. Breathe in through your nose, and exhale through your nose.

Week 9 – Exercise 18 Laugh Lines
(Gloves are required)

All areas of your face and neck have been well exercised throughout the past several weeks. The last exercise addresses your upper cheeks from a different perspective, and the muscles that surround the lower portion of your face will also contract.

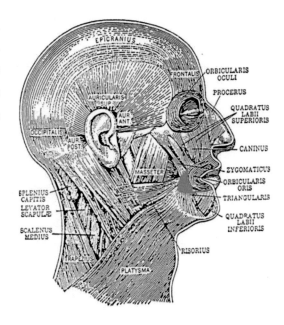

Left side

1. Insert your right thumb into the left side of your mouth, and place it under your laugh line, about one inch from the corner of your mouth. This is located at the junction of the Zygomaticus (cheek muscle) and the Orbicularis Oris (mouth muscle).

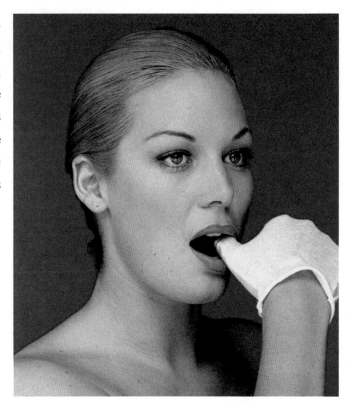

2. Curve your index finger over your laugh line on the outside of your face.
3. **Grip** the laugh line firmly between your thumb and your index finger.
4. Open your mouth wide and gently pull the corner of your mouth straight towards the center of your mouth to make your muscle taut.
5. Hold the muscle in place and then **contract** it by trying to pull the corner of your mouth towards your ear. Hold the contraction for five (5) seconds.

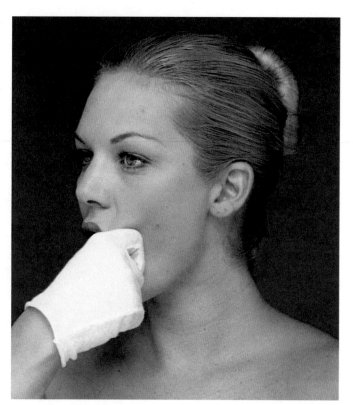

6. Remove your hand from your face.
7. Breathe in deeply through your nose, and exhale through your nose.
8. Repeat the three remaining sets, holding the contractions for ten (10) seconds each.
9. Breathe in deeply through your nose, and exhale through your nose.

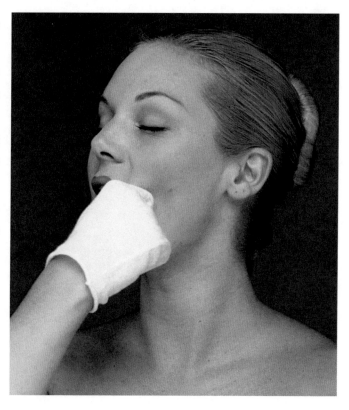

Right side

1. Insert your left thumb into the right side of your mouth and place it under your laugh line about one inch from the corner of your mouth.

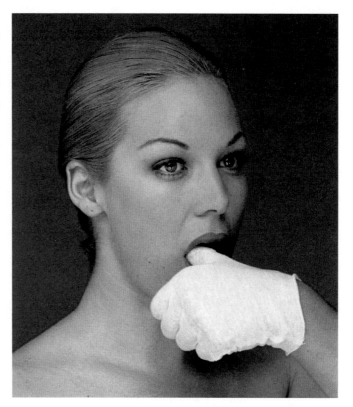

2. Curve your index finger over your laugh line on the outside of your face.

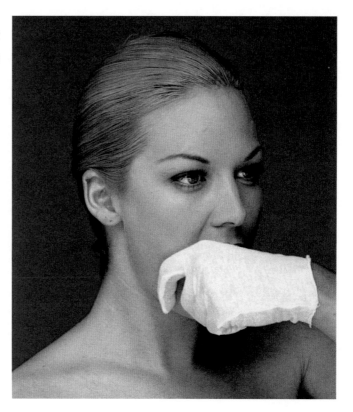

3. **Grip** the laugh line firmly between your thumb and your index finger.

4. Open your mouth wide and gently pull the corner of your mouth straight towards the center of your mouth to make your muscle taut.

5. Hold the muscle in place and then contract it by trying to pull the corner of your mouth towards your ear. Hold the contraction for five (5) seconds.

6. Remove your hand from your face.

7. Breathe in deeply through your nose, and exhale through your nose.

8. Repeat the three remaining sets, holding the contractions for ten (10) seconds each.

9. Breathe in deeply through your nose, and exhale through your nose.

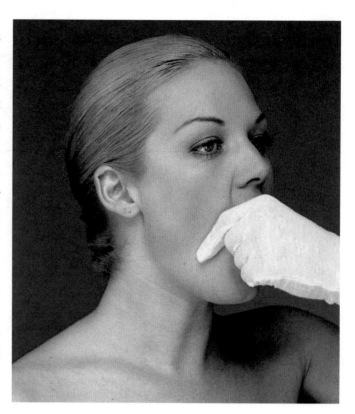

Week Nine Affirmations:
Each day is my opportunity to experience the beauty of life.
I look for beauty today in myself and in my friends.
I absorb the brilliance of life!

Chapter Twenty-Three – Luscious Lips

Lips - Bardot lips, Angelina lips. Full, pouty, sexy lips. Traffic stopping lips. Have you noticed that your lips are shrinking and not as full as they were when you were in your twenties? You may realize that in your late 30's and early 40's you have lost volume in your face and in your lips. Facial Magic will plump up the facial muscles so that you look younger, but what about your lips? Is there anything that can restore those full, pouty lips you had when you were younger?

Yes there is! Luscious Lips, a hand held device, is ideal to restore youthful, fuller lips. The device provides a natural way to enhance your lips as it increases your lip size quickly, easily and safely. The results will be exactly what you wanted!

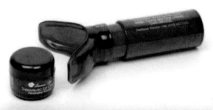

When your lips lose volume, you may see lines developing that result in lipstick bleed lines. These lines will continue to develop if left unchecked. You may stop wearing lipstick altogether rather than run the risk of wearing embarrassing lipstick streaks that creep into every crevice.

Let me share my story with you. I had been asked to have new headshots taken and when I looked at the many pages of contact sheets, I noticed that something was "different" about my face. My skin was taut, my eyes were open but there was something wrong! After days of scrutiny, I discovered that the difference I was seeing was in my lips. My top lip particularly looked shrunken and I did not like that look. I felt that the loss of volume was disturbing and if I continued to lose volume, I would have no apparent top lip over time. After months of research, Luscious Lips was born.

The Luscious Lips device is small and can fit easily and discreetly into most purses. How does it work? The specially designed mouthpiece creates a vacuum that draws fluid to your lips from the surrounding tissue. The result is fuller lips in just seconds a day.

When you first begin using the device, you must "condition" your lips for 10-14 days; this means that you should use the device sparingly to slowly introduce the fluid into your lips again. In fact, you should use the device only ten seconds per day for five two-second intervals. This action is ideal for bringing fluid to your lips. After the initial conditioning period, your lips will be ready to become fuller by using the device for twenty to thirty seconds per day.

You can choose the volume that suits your face best. Some users (both men and women enjoy this little red device) feel that a twenty to thirty second plump is perfect for daytime. The results will last for hours as long as you correctly "condition" your lips. For nighttime, you may want to create "Hollywood" lips, very full, pouty lips. If that is your desire, you may want to use the device for three twenty second pulls for a total of sixty seconds.

Using the device is painless, takes just seconds to use and is affordable.

The results produced by Luscious Lips look natural. No bumps or lumps, just smooth, hydrated, kissable lips. You will love how it enhances your smile! It is truly a "face saving" method of correcting one of Mother Nature's foibles.

Luscious Lips was featured on Rachael Ray's "Human Lab," the Tonight Show with Jay Leno, The Doctors and Donnie & Marie. The "Price is Right" girls loved it.

FACIAL MAGIC®

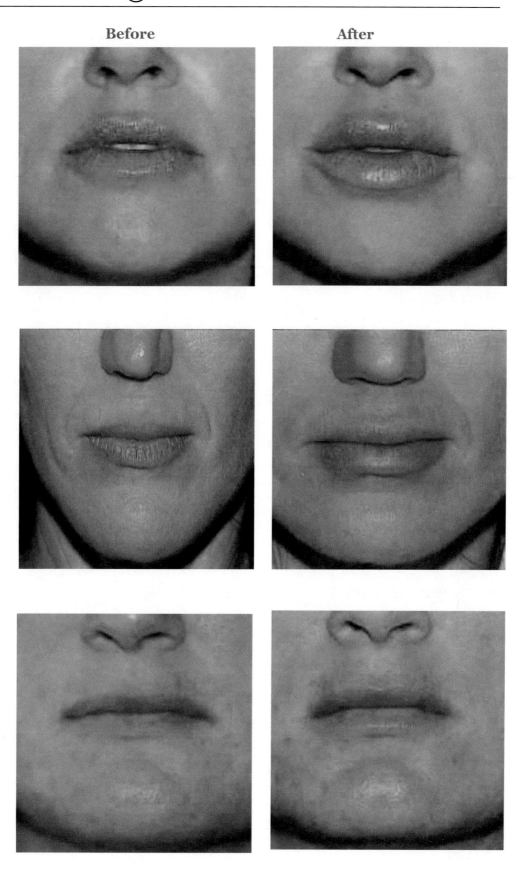

Therapeutic Lip Crème

To accompany the Luscious Lips device, we have developed our own special Therapeutic Lip Crème that hydrates and even increases the plump.

As you mature, you find dry skin apparent around your mouth and lips. The Luscious Lips Therapeutic Lip Crème is not only an effective treatment for the lips themselves, it is also specially formulated for the skin (tissue) surrounding the lips. This sensitive area is one of the first places that the signs of aging begin to appear. These are usually seen as fine lines and creases around your mouth accompanied by a loss of tone (firmness) and elasticity. This specially designed crème can be used both day and night. Therapeutic Lip Crème can be used alone, or under balms, gloss or lipstick.

Benefits

Moisturizing and Increased Plumping

The Therapeutic Lip Crème moisturizes the lips and surrounding areas leaving them soft and supple. Increasing the moisture level also plumps the skin to reduce the appearance of fine lines and wrinkles, while at the same time, increasing the skin's firmness and elasticity to help avoid the formation of new lines and creases. The formula includes Sepi-Lift, an ingredient from France that enhances and increases the moisture binding properties.

Anti-Oxidants

The Therapeutic Lip Creme has been formulated with two highly effective anti-oxidants: Vitamin E and Vitamin C. These two primary ingredients help smooth, protect and moisturize the skin while helping to protect the skin against free radicals.

Vitamin C is known to stimulate the cells of the dermis in the production of collagen and elastin and other components of the Intercellular Matrix. All of these materials are very important to health of the skin and enable it to combat the signs of aging.

Frequently Asked Questions About Luscious Lips

The Luscious Lips Device

Q. How does Luscious Lips work?

A. Luscious Lips uses a natural vacuum process to draw fluid from around the mouth area into the lips, plumping the lips and increasing circulation in the lip and mouth area.

Q. What is the two-week conditioning period?

A. In the beginning, the tissue in the lips is not prepared to receive large volumes of additional fluid. By using the device sparingly the first two weeks, your lip tissue will be gradually enhanced. We recommend five two-second "pulls" per day for the first two weeks. After the initial two-week conditioning period, increase the duration of the "pulls" to five seconds for a few days. Following this conditioning routine will minimize bruising or discoloration of the lips that can result from over zealous users. Do not exceed two minutes in total (4 thirty-second pulls).

Q. What should I do if I get a bruise on my lips?

A. Bruising should not occur if the conditioning process is carefully followed. If you experience bruising or discoloration, stop using the device until the bruise goes away. Then, begin the conditioning process again to gradually build up the tissue in the lips to receive the additional fluid.

Q. How long does the plump last?

A. Results will vary with each individual. The duration of the plump will depend on your personal metabolism and the duration of the "pulls." For example, three twenty-second pulls will create fuller lips for a longer period of time than 3 ten-second pulls. Most women report that a "medium plump" will last 4-8 hours. We recommend that you create a medium plump in the morning and plump again during the day as needed.

Q. How long does it take each day?

A. Following the initial conditioning period, Luscious Lips works in just a few seconds each time. Experienced users can achieve a "Hollywood" plump with 3 thirty-second pulls, a total of 90 seconds. In general, we recommend that pulls do not exceed twenty seconds and that total time does not exceed 120 seconds.

Q. Can I use Luscious Lips more than once a day?

A. YES! Most women find that using the Luscious Lips device several times a day keeps their lips plump and full. We recommend several medium plumps each day rather than one prolonged plump.

Q. Is it safe?

A. YES. Doctor supervised studies have determined that Luscious Lips is safe and effective when used as directed. Because the results are temporary, there are no long-term effects from using Luscious Lips.

Q. Am I too old to use Luscious Lips?

A. NO. Many women in their 70's and 80's have found Luscious Lips to be effective in counteracting the shrinking of the lips that naturally occurs with loss of volume in the face due to aging.

Q. Will Luscious Lips help reduce the appearance of fine lines on and around my lips?

A. Most women report that fine lines around the lips are diminished with continued use of the Luscious Lips device and the Therapeutic Lip Crème.

Q. Does using the device hurt?

A. NO! The process should never be painful. When using the Luscious Lips device, allow the device to gently draw the lips into the mouthpiece, hold for a few seconds, and release the vacuum. It is not necessary to pull the vacuum to its maximum power to achieve the desired results.

Q. I have a narrow face. Will Luscious Lips work for me?

A. The mouthpiece of the Luscious Lips device has been designed to accommodate the facial shape of most women. Women with narrow faces sometimes have difficulty achieving an airtight seal around the mouthpiece, which is necessary to create the vacuum. Usually, turning the device upside down and positioning the "bottom" of the mouthpiece just under the nose can remedy this situation.

Q. Can I use Luscious Lips if I have dental work (bridges, plates, etc.)?

A. Using the Luscious Lips device will have no effect on dental work.

Q. I have had collagen injections in the past. Can I still use Luscious Lips?

A. Luscious Lips is ideal for women who have had collagen injections in the past. Even women who are currently receiving collagen injections find that the use of Luscious Lips helps to smooth the lumps caused from collagen injections.

Q. I have had thin lips all my life. Will Luscious Lips work for me?

A. Luscious Lips works to increase the size and plumpness of lips of all sizes. You should expect to achieve up to 50% increase in volume of your lips.

Q. I am a mature person and am taking blood-thinning medication. Should I use Luscious Lips?

A. Check with your doctor. Blood thinning medication can make you more susceptible to bruising and Luscious Lips may not be for you. Also, if you are prone to cold sores or bruise easily, you may not be able to use Luscious Lips.

Frequently Asked Questions: Therapeutic Lip Crème

Q. What makes the Therapeutic Lip Crème so special?

A. Vitamin C, Vitamin E, Macadamia Nut Oil and collagen. The Vitamin C and Vitamin E are highly effective anti-oxidants that attack oxidants, also known as free radicals. Free radicals are very damaging to skin cells and are considered one of the leading causes of premature aging. The Macadamia Nut Oil was chosen for its exceptional emollient qualities. It is very rich in Essential Fatty Acids that help to combat dry skin conditions. Collagen adds structure to the intercellular matrix of the skin and helps replace natural collagen lost due to aging. The combination of these ingredients penetrates the sensitive skin of the lips and mouth area to hydrate the tissue, firming the skin and reducing the appearance of the fine vertical lines.

Q. **When should I use Therapeutic Lip Crème?**

A. Apply TLC to clean skin in the morning under makeup and again at bedtime.

Q. **Do I use Therapeutic Lip Crème at the same time as the Luscious Lips device?**

A. TLC complements the plumping effects of the Luscious Lips device, but is used independently. Use TLC in the morning under makeup and again at bedtime. Use the Luscious Lips device at least once a day to maintain the condition of the lip tissue.

Maintenance

Q. **How do I clean my Luscious Lips device?**

A. Do not immerse the device in water. Simply wipe the device with a paper towel lightly dampened with a mild cleaning solution.

Now enjoy reading the following testimonials and seeing before and after photos from a few of my friends.

Chapter Twenty-Four – Testimonials

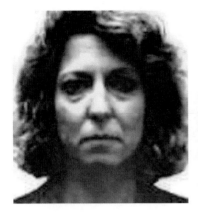 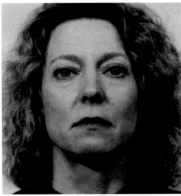 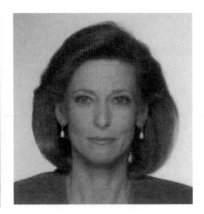

My name is Diann Kaufmann and I love what Facial Magic has done for me. One day I caught a glimpse of myself in the mirror and realized just how much I was beginning to resemble my mother. Do not get me wrong, I love my Mother, but at 48, I did not want to look like her.

Then I began to seem invisible to the opposite sex, and my confidence left me. About that time, a brochure arrived at my home describing a non-surgical method of correcting the areas of my face that concerned me; my cheeks were spongy, jowls were beginning to form and worst of all, I knew people saw the bags under my eyes first. I kept that brochure around for days, reading and re-reading the text, and it all began to make sense to me. I had a feeling these specialized exercises for the face would work for me.

I began the Facial Magic program and in a matter of days, I saw subtle changes in my face. In weeks my upper cheeks began to develop in such a way that I had "high cheekbones". (The bones had been there all the time but my sagging muscles prevented a more youthful look.) At the end of eleven weeks my entire face was firm, lifted and toned; most importantly, the bags under my eyes were gone! Facial Magic gave me a much younger appearance and I will use it for the rest of my life!

FACIAL MAGIC- "I am living proof that the exercises have helped me feel better a\bout myself and that they do work."

You have a great product. I am 43 and teach at SFSU - so I am around very young & very old people. When I tell my students my age... (yes, the little buggers do ask)...they are often surprised. *Patti, California*

LUSCIOUS LIPS- "Give it a try."

Skeptical at first. I now know the Luscious Lips Pump has made my lips beautiful and definitely made fine lines around my mouth disappear. Give it a try! *Helen, Ontario, Canada*

LUSCIOUS LIPS - "Thank you for making a dream come true."

I am absolutely amazed at the results I had from using this device! It REALLY works! I am elated! I have wished for full lips since I was a little girl. I would not hesitate to recommend this to anyone. Thank you so much for making a dream come true. *Rosalind, Birmingham*

LUSCIOUS LIPS - "...nothing makes lips as sensual and youthful looking."

We would just like to say, as two really cool chicks, that for any woman (or man) who doesn't want to take the route of injection, NOTHING, and we mean NOTHING, makes lips as sensual and youthful looking (no matter what your age) as does the Lip Pump. Thank you! *Babs & Reetz, Ontario, Canada*

FACIAL MAGIC - "Facial Magic has enriched my life."

The results I see in my face of firmness and texture truly give me a more youthful appearance. I love being part of the success of this product, for the integrity and truth for what it claims, but... most of all, I LOVE Cynthia Rowland. Her commitment to her program, together with her encouragement and dedication combine to make a youthful face possible for everyone. Yeah, Facial Magic! And, Yeah, Cynthia Rowland. *Nancy O., Santa Monica, CA.*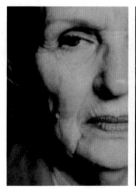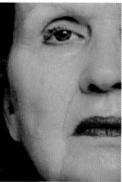

FACIAL MAGIC - "I love it and it certainly does work."

I have been using your Facial Magic system for about three years. I just love it and it certainly does work. Thank you. *Joan W., Meaford, Ont. Canada*

FACIAL MAGIC®

LUSCIOUS LIPS - "...my lips [look] fuller and younger."

Dear Cynthia, I wanted to let you know how much I love the Luscious Lips device. I am 54 and my l;ips look younger, fuller and more defined. I would recommend it to anyone. I have two daughters in their middle twenties and they both noticed that my lips looked fuller and younger. Thank you, *Maria J. Hermitage, Tennessee*

FACIAL MAGIC - "My hanging chin is gone."

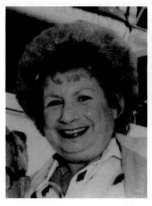 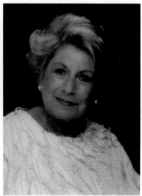

I am extremely pleased at what I see in the mirror when I look at my face. Lines along my forehead have disappeared. I can now see eye shadow between my eyelid and eye brow which I have not seen in years. It looks like I had an eyelift. My cheeks have plumped up near my eyes and heavy lines near my eyes are less. My hanging chin is gone. I can see a jaw line. When a neighbor of mine recently asked me if I had a facelift, I knew I was doing something right. Thanks for bringing Facial magic to me. It has given me more esteem than I have ever had. *Bernice U. Tamarac, FL*

LUSCIOUS LIPS - "...I really do not think I could live without it now."

I really like the lip pump, and it gives my lips a much fuller and supple appearance. I use it in the morning before I put on my lipstick and it adds a lot more definition and fullness. My husband can really tell the difference. For anyone who has ever been self conscious of their lips or mouth it makes you feel confident. Thanks...I really do not think I could live without it now. *Kelly*

LUSCIOUS LIPS - "I love the way my lips look after using the pump."

I have been using the lip pump for a couple months now and the results are great. I have had collagen injections before but they do not last and they are very expensive. The pump makes the lines around my mouth plump out & become hardly noticeable. I love the way my lips look after using the pump. Thank you, Thank you. *Barbara L. Fremont, CA*

LUSCIOUS LIPS - "...the change in the size of my lips is incredible."

I have had the lip pump for about three months now, and the change in the size of my lips is incredible. I have always been self-conscious about having what I perceive to be thin lips, and have found the Lip Pump to be safe, quick, and with results that last for the whole workday. I feel a lot better about myself - a lot more attractive - and recommend this product to ANY woman who would like fuller lips but is wary of collagen injections and other more invasive procedures. Thank you very much for creating this product! *Barbara V. Toronto, Ontario Canada*

LUSCIOUS LIPS - "UNBELIEVABLE"

As a makeup artist and former representative for a world-renowned cosmetic company, I feel confident in stating that there is nothing in the cosmetic marketplace that can enlarge the lips and help make fine lines around the mouth disappear (albeit temporarily) to the degree that the Lip Pump can. In brief: It has to be tried to be believed - UNBELIEVABLE, but it is believable, because I tried it, and it works. *Rita H., Toronto, Ontario, Canada*

LUSCIOUS LIPS - "...I can achieve really full, pouty lips when I want."

The lip pump device has been wonderful for me. I have never liked my thin lips and was tired of the expense and pain of collagen injections. My next step was going to be surgery before I heard about the lip pump. After several weeks of following the directions, I began to notice my lips looking much fuller. Now after using the device for several months I can achieve really full, pouty lips when I want. If you want full lips without the expense and pain of surgery please give the lip pump a try. I think you will be glad you did. *Monya*

LUSCIOUS LIPS - "I love Luscious Lips.."

I received the lip pump in the mail yesterday, and want to thank you very much for your help with my lip pump emergency! I have my device and feel human again (what does that say about me?). Anyway, thanks again. I love Luscious Lips and am telling all my girlfriends about it, and some of the guys too, though they just give me weird looks. Best regards, *Barbara V., Toronto*

Chapter Twenty-Five – Before & After

In the fourteen years since I began instructing Facial Magic clients, I have seen the incredible transformations of their faces. Some have called the amazing lifting and toning "miracles".

Along with the testimonials and before and after photographs in Chapter 24, I would now like to show you more remarkable results obtained by another six Facial Magic clients.

You can see from their ages, the rejuvenation process can begin at any time and works for every face!

These women took the challenge and made the commitment to improve their appearance and self-confidence. They took control of the aging process, met it "face-on" and never looked back. The simplicity of the exercises, the build up of muscle tone seen from week to week allowed them to make Facial Magic a way of life, something you do automatically every day, like brushing your teeth or taking a shower.

Having now completed the System, I am sure that your before and after photos are as dramatic as these. I would love to see your photographs and read your testimonials. Please send letters and photos to: *cynthia@cynthiarowland.com.*

Betty W. had a common problem; she had developed a matronly jaw line at the tender age of 48. Her upper cheeks were indistinguishable and her jowls were prominent. In eight weeks she had significantly toned the lower portion of her face and as a result, she appears more youthful.

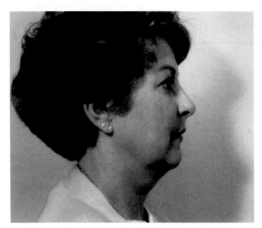 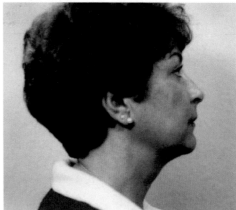

At age 48, Darlene D. wanted a toned, fresh look and in eight weeks, you can see that her jowl area and posture are much improved. Her cheeks appear lifted and her neck and nose are more defined.

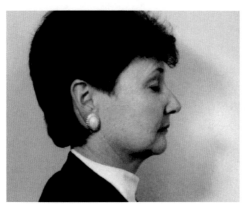 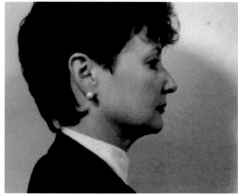

Victoria T. at age 48 wanted to get rid of the slackness she saw developing under her chin. In nine weeks her cheeks lifted, her upper eye area improved and her chin became sculpted and toned.

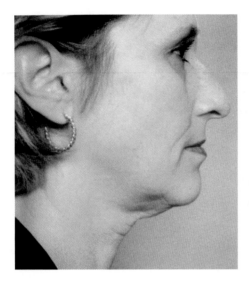 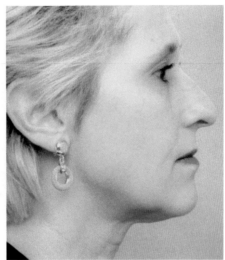

Inge C. is an actress and she loves her new look. Her pouches and cheek areas had become slack and her neck had lost its tone. In a few weeks she saw amazing tightening in those areas and her entire face smoothed, toned and lifted.

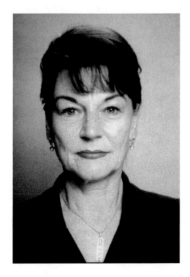 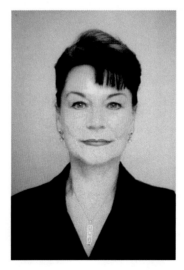

Lillian H., the former Mrs. Colorado, dramatically improved her face, neck and posture in just twelve weeks. Notice how her head is youthfully positioned and how toned and vibrant her face is.

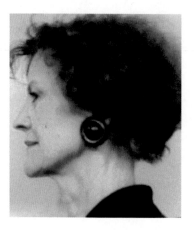 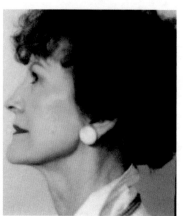

Her eyes are open and she is rejuvenated! She does not look 63!

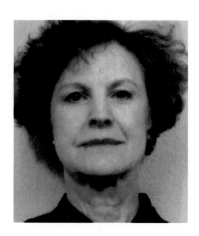 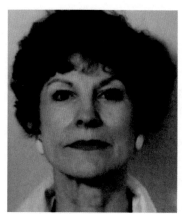

Shirley D. certainly doesn't look 48 in her before picture does she? Her face and neck showed severe aging and her skin looked unhealthy. In twelve weeks, there is great improvement; her jaw line has revitalized and her upper eyes have lifted. She looks so wonderful!

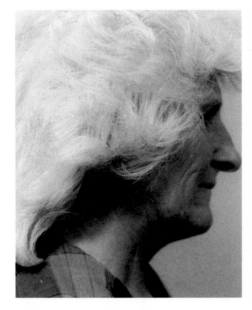 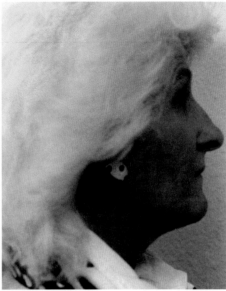

Chapter Twenty-Six – In Closing…

Writing this book has given me great satisfaction. Knowing that you can now take control of your face with these natural, proven methods to keep you looking as young as you feel, makes me proud.

I wish I could stand beside you while you perform each movement because nothing gives me greater pleasure than to watch a Facial Magic user transform his or her face. You can do this! You can take charge of your facial appearance to make it more beautiful and alluring with these exercises, so do not hesitate to begin this very easy process of facial rehabilitation. You will be so proud of yourself and your accomplishments!

Our training classes and programs are available on DVD and online at *www.cynthiarowland.com*.

Index